Ultrasound Protocol for Facial Aesthetics

Kathryn Malherbe • Stefania Roberts

Ultrasound Protocol for Facial Aesthetics

A practical clinical guide

Springer

Kathryn Malherbe
Malherbe Imaging Inc
Diagnostic Imaging Solutions
Pretoria, South Africa

Stefania Roberts
Victoria Vein Clinic
East Melbourne, VIC, Australia

ISBN 978-3-031-75948-2 ISBN 978-3-031-75949-9 (eBook)
https://doi.org/10.1007/978-3-031-75949-9

This Springer imprint is published by the registered company Springer Nature Switzerland AG
The registered company address is: Gewerbestrasse 11, 6330 Cham, Switzerland

Contents

List of Figures

1 Introduction

High-frequency ultrasound, predominantly used in radiology, has progressed in recent years to other fields of medicine, most notably aesthetic medicine. Facial ultrasound, previously limited to the clinical assessment of varying dermatological conditions, has now gained increased acceptance and use as a valuable tool in day to day clinical practice by aesthetic clinicians to identify the layers of the face, previously injected filler materials, to locate important vascular structures and to assist during aesthetic treatments [1].

The importance of ultrasound protocols in medical imaging cannot be overstated. These standardized sets of procedures and guidelines play a pivotal role in ensuring consistency, accuracy, and efficiency throughout ultrasound examinations. By providing a systematic framework for imaging practices, protocols promote uniformity across different healthcare providers and settings. This not only enhances the quality of imaging but also facilitates easy comparisons of images over time [1–6]. The efficiency gained from following established protocols is particularly valuable in busy clinical environments, enabling quick and accurate diagnostics. Moreover, protocols contribute to quality assurance by minimizing variability, reducing the likelihood of errors, and serving as valuable tools for education and training of ultrasound practitioners. This standardized approach supports informed clinical decision-making, improves patient care by enhancing diagnostic precision, and fosters research and audit activities, ultimately advancing medical knowledge and improving overall healthcare quality. In essence, ultrasound protocols are integral to the modern practice of medical imaging, ensuring a structured and consistent approach to diagnostic examinations [1–6].

An ultrasound protocol refers to a systematic and standardized set of procedures, techniques, and guidelines followed during an ultrasound examination. It serves as a structured framework designed to ensure consistency, accuracy, and efficiency in acquiring diagnostic images. Ultrasound protocols are specific to different anatomical regions or clinical indications, outlining the necessary steps, imaging planes, and parameters to be considered during the examination [1, 7, 8].

An ultrasound protocol requires the following systematic parameters to be used optimally in practice:

- Patient preparation, such as removal of clothing or jewelry that may interfere with imaging.
- Identify the appropriate transducer type and frequency based on the target anatomy, depth of structures, and the clinical question at hand.
- Optimal placement of the ultrasound probe on the patient's body, including specific anatomical landmarks and imaging planes to be utilized.

K. Malherbe, S. Roberts, *Ultrasound Protocol for Facial Aesthetics*,
https://doi.org/10.1007/978-3-031-75949-9_1

- Outline ultrasound machine settings, including gain, depth, focal zones, and any specific adjustments required to optimize image quality for the examination.
- Specify any dynamic maneuver or patient position that may aid in visualizing specific structures or assessing functional aspects during the examination.
- Detail the required images or video clips to be captured, ensuring comprehensive coverage of the relevant anatomical structures and pathology.
- Provide guidance on the interpretation of ultrasound findings, including criteria for normal and abnormal appearances, measurements, and potential diagnostic considerations.

The past 10 years have seen a dramatic increase of non-surgical aesthetic treatments with the most recent published Aesthetics Society And Plastic Surgery (ASAP) data of 2021 [9, 10] showing an overall increase of facial procedures by 55%. This increase in non-surgical aesthetic treatments has led to a rising number of complications and poor clinical outcomes. The increased use of neurotoxin from 2020 has been reported as 40%, dermal fillers increased by 43% in both male and female patients between the ages of 38–50 years. The highest increase, however, was in the reversal of dermal fillers which was reported by ASAP as 69%. Latest statistics of ASAP in 2022, has shown that from pre pandemic era (2019) to 2022, there has been a steady increase in the use of neuromodulator injections, averaging at 73% since 2019 [9–11]. Hyaluronic acid (HA) fillers also showed from 2019–2022, a 70% increase in use. The Top 5 Minimally Invasive Procedures for 2022 was stated as: Neuromodulator injections, Soft tissue HA fillers, Skin resurfacing, Skin treatments and lastly lip augmentation [9–11].

The popularity of videoconferencing platforms skyrocketed during the COVID-19 pandemic; with video calls promoting dissatisfaction and dysmorphism of the observers facial appearance, termed the so-called "Zoom effect" [12]. This phenomenon has contributed to the rising increase of body dissatisfaction and body dysmorphism associated with facial aesthetics and the rising incidence of its use in clinical practice. The psychological impact of aesthetic treatments is key and however, not within the scope of this book. Aesthetic medicine is performed by a range of practitioners worldwide with differing skill sets and formal training programs. When performing injectable facial treatments, relying solely on surface anatomy and anatomical knowledge from medical texts, or even attending and performing cadaver dissections of the face, is insufficient for accurately assessing the potential risks associated with facial injectable treatments, particularly when it comes to inadvertent arterial injection. It is imperative to recognize these limitations and seek out more comprehensive methods of evaluation to ensure the safety and well-being of patients [12].

For this reason, ultrasound of the face has allowed clinicians to develop a keen sense of vascular presence in real-time at the bedside prior to treatments, assessment of facial musculature, in addition to determining the depth when performing ultrasound guided injections. Ultrasound allows visualization of previous filler, as part of the initial assessment, when a patient presents to the clinician for the first and subsequent visits.

Patients are presenting to their clinicians armed with more information and knowledge, not necessarily evidence based, due to the rise of multiple social media platforms. As a result, the patients are also finding the use of ultrasound during aesthetic treatment as the so-called "awe phenomenon," as the combination of aesthetic appearance and sonographic confirmation of the aesthetic intervention develops a trust factor between the patient and the doctor, thereby optimizing the overall outcome [10, 11, 13].

This book aims to provide a systematic approach to facial ultrasound, using anatomical surface landmarks to assist the clinician when performing aesthetic facial treatment. It also includes the most common clinical indications and complications found during aesthetic therapy.

References

1. Wu WT, Chang KV, Chang HC, Chen LR, Kuan CH, Kao JT, et al. Ultrasound imaging of the facial muscles and relevance with Botulinum toxin injections: a pictorial essay and narrative review. Toxins (Basel). 2022;14(2) https://doi.org/10.3390/toxins14020101.

2. Zetlaoui PJ, Gauthier E, Benhamou D. Ultrasound-guided scalp nerve blocks for neurosurgery: a narrative review. Anaesth Crit Care Pain Med. 2020;39(6):876–82. https://doi.org/10.1016/j.accpm.2020.06.019.
3. Bhoi S, Chandra A, Galwankar S. Ultrasound-guided nerve blocks in the emergency department. J Emerg Trauma Shock. 2010;3(1):82–8. https://doi.org/10.4103/0974-2700.58655.
4. Ryu JH, Shim JH, Yeom JH, Shin WJ, Cho SY, Jeon WJ. Ultrasound-guided greater occipital nerve block with botulinum toxin for patients with chronic headache in the occipital area: a randomized controlled trial. Korean J Anesthesiol. 2019;72(5):479–85. https://doi.org/10.4097/kja.19145.
5. Kim SH. Interpretation of peripheral arterial and venous Doppler waveforms: a consensus statement from the Society for Vascular Medicine and Society for vascular ultrasound. Vasc Med. 2020;25(5):484–506.
6. Gerr A [Internet]. Anisotropy as most important pitfall in ultrasound imaging. 2023. Available from: www.sonoskills.com.
7. Food and Drug Administration. XEOMIN (incobotulinumtoxinA). Silver Spring, MD: FDA; 2010. p. 10.
8. Food and Drug Administration. BOTOX (onabotulinumtoxinA). In: Drug FM, editor. FDA; 1989.
9. Greco GA. Plastic surgery statistics report. Arlington Heights, IL: American Soceity of Plastic Surgeons; 2022.
10. The Aesthetic Soceity. The aesthetic society statistics. Aesthetic Plastic Surgery National Databank, 2021.
11. Sundaram H, Signorini M, Liew S, Trindade de Almeida AR, Wu Y, Vieira Braz A, et al. Global Aesthetics Consensus: Botulinum Toxin Type A--Evidence-Based Review, Emerging Concepts, and Consensus Recommendations for Aesthetic Use, Including Updates on Complications. Plast Reconstr Surg 2016; 137(3):518e-529e. https://doi.org/10.1097/01.prs.0000475758.63709.23.
12. Pikoos TD, Buzwell S, Sharp G, Rossell SL. The zoom effect: exploring the impact of video calling on appearance dissatisfaction and interest in aesthetic treatment during the COVID-19 pandemic. Aesthet Surg J. 2021;41(12):NP2066–75. https://doi.org/10.1093/asj/sjab257.
13. Samizadeh S, De Boulle K. Complications of toxins and fillers in facial aesthetics. Prim Dent J. 2023;12(3):65–72.

Sonographic Principles and Techniques

2

In the realm of facial aesthetics, ultrasound techniques have emerged as indispensable tools for non-invasive imaging, providing clinicians with valuable insights into the intricate structures and dynamics of facial tissues. Utilizing ultrasound imaging, practitioners can explore the facial anatomy in various planes, capturing detailed cross-sectional views that contribute to a comprehensive understanding of tissue composition and vascularization. Furthermore, dynamic techniques, such as real-time imaging and Doppler assessments, add an extra dimension by allowing clinicians to observe tissue movement, perfusion patterns, and vascular dynamics, enhancing the precision of facial aesthetic procedures and optimizing patient outcomes.

The ultrasound transducer to be used for facial aesthetics is the linear transducer with a frequency of at least 15 MhZ and above to ensure optimal resolution.

The transducer orientation is in two main planes, namely longitudinal and transverse. In certain anatomical planes an oblique approach can be used:

Longitudinal refers to the section being imaged in a sagittal anatomical plane (Fig. 2.1), seeing the structures on the ultrasound image from superior to inferior [1–6].

Transverse refers to the section being imaged in an axial anatomical plane, seeing the structures on the ultrasound image from lateral to medial (Fig. 2.2)

The transducer has an anatomical orientation notch which allows the user to place either the most superior or most lateral portion on the left side of the screen (Fig. 2.3).

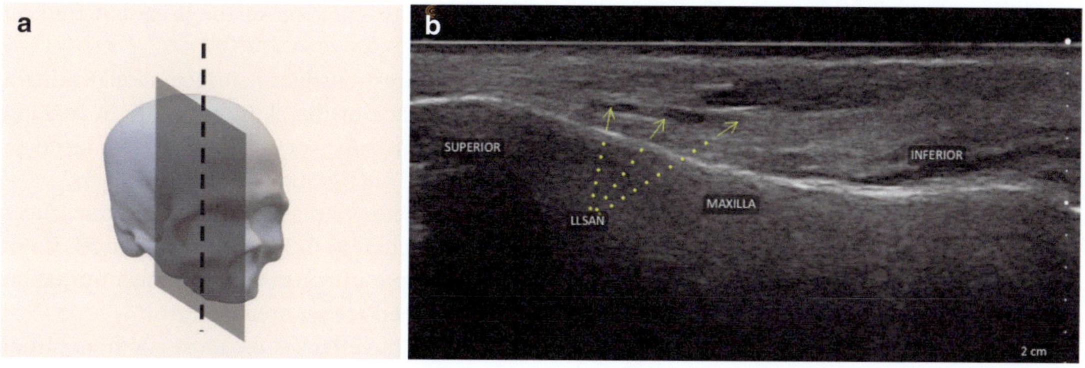

Fig. 2.1 Longitudinal plane on ultrasound. (**a**) Depiction of sagittal plane of the skull. (**b**) Sonographic depiction of sagittal plane as presented in (**a**)

K. Malherbe, S. Roberts, *Ultrasound Protocol for Facial Aesthetics*,
https://doi.org/10.1007/978-3-031-75949-9_2

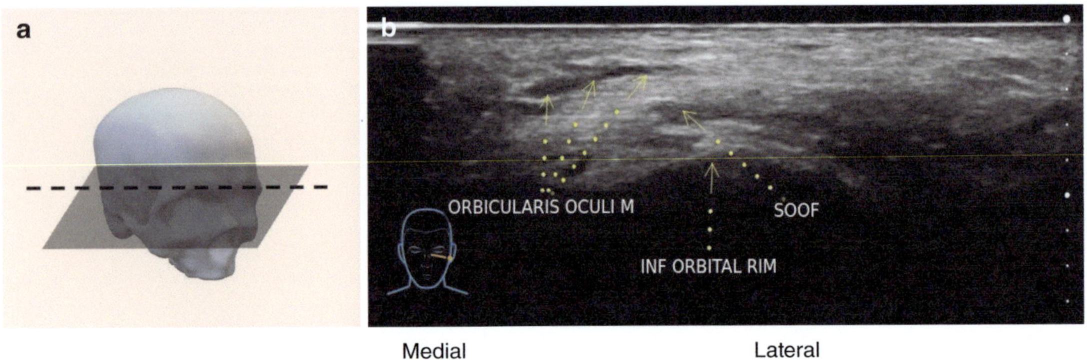

Fig. 2.2 Transverse plane on ultrasound. (**a**) Depiction of the transverse or axial plane of the skull. (**b**) Sonographic depiction of transverse plane as presented in (**a**)

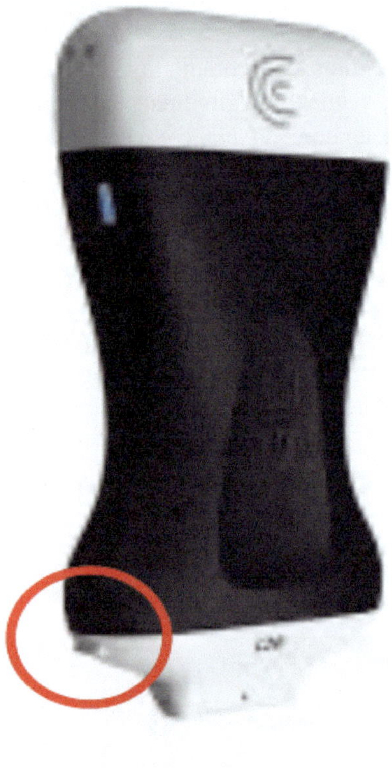

Fig. 2.3 Orientation marker
Orientation marker on the ultrasound probe (red circle) indicates the direction of the ultrasound image
Transverse plane, the marker is directed to the left side
Sagittal plane, the marker is directed to the superior edge

2.1 Ultrasound Techniques During Imaging

Using the orientation marker, the "heel-toe" method can be used to opt for a systematic approach to sonographic imaging.

This refers to keeping the orientation marker (the heel) on a fixed anatomical landmark and only moving the opposite end of the transducer surface (the toe) in a different direction.

The heel toe method can be used for areas such as the curved mentum, the tear trough and the nasolabial fold. The heel toe method (Fig. 2.4) is also often used for sweeping from medial to lateral in the tear trough to determine the presence of the angular artery and vein.

Heel toe is commonly used to tilt the angle of insonance to the vessel of interest (Fig. 2.5), through slight compression of the heel or toe portion of the transducer [7, 9–13].

The face is composed of a series of curved surfaces, so called O-gee curves, advised to apply slight rocking, or tilting of the transducer along the curved surface to ensure a true anatomical representation of the area depicted on ultrasound.

The entire transducer surface should remain on the surface of the skin, and a slight rocking motion from superior to inferior is induced to enhance the sonographic output (Fig. 2.6).

It is imperative that the ultrasound transducer is perpendicular to the anatomy of interest, if not an anisotropic effect may cause misinformation of the planned area of treatment.

Anisotropic effect is the most common pitfall reported during use of B-mode ultrasound with a linear transducer. It refers to the sonographic darkening and loss of resolution when the approach of sound waves is not perpendicular (less than 0°) to the area of interest [6].

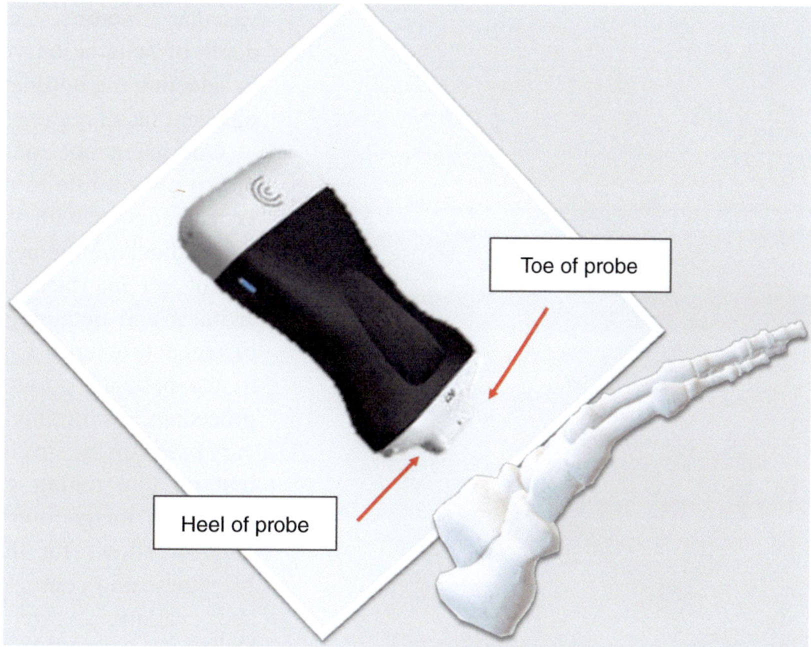

Fig. 2.4 Heel and toe method
Heel and toe refers to the orientation marker representing the "heel" of the foot, which remains stationary, and the opposite edge of the toe of the probe representing the motion to left or right whilst the heel remains in position

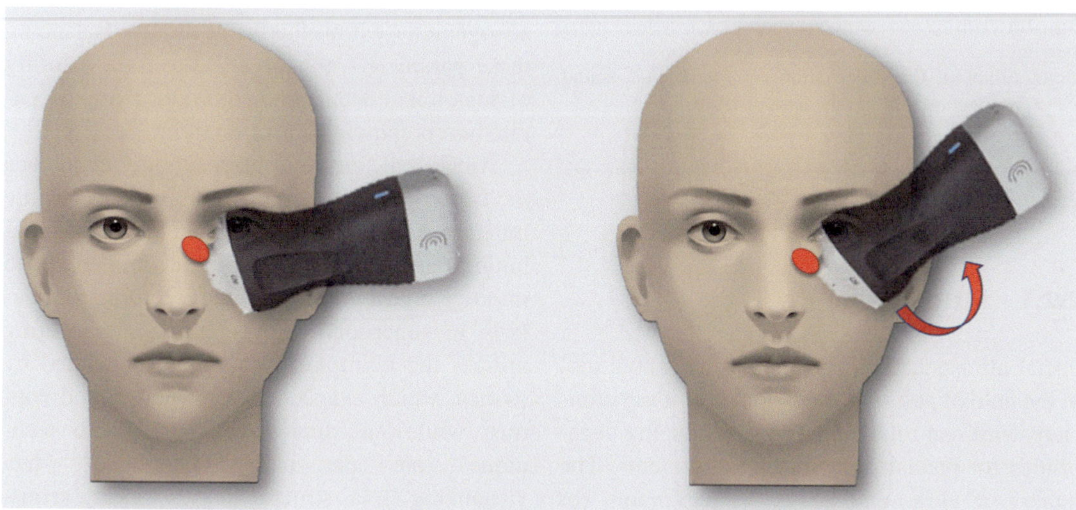

Fig. 2.5 Heel and toe method for sonographic imaging of the angular artery and vein
Image left: Position 1: Heel remains on the medial canthus of the left eye (red dot). Toe is aligned along the nasolabial fold
Image right: Position 2: Heel remains on the medial canthus of the left eye (red dot). Toe is rotated lateral towards the maxilla (curved arrow)

Another method is to make use of a gel stand-off pad to simulate an even skin surface when a curved underlying structure is impeding optimal imaging output.

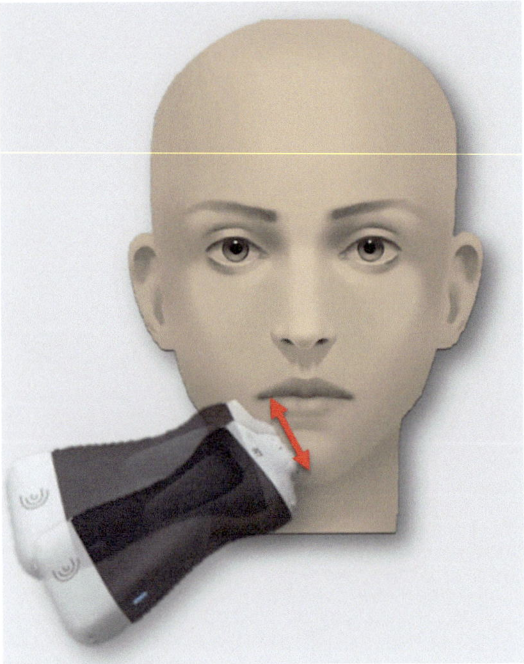

Fig. 2.6 Tilting and angling method for sonographic imaging
Slight tilting of the probe allows perpendicular sound wave propogation through the area of interest

2.2 Image Optimization During Facial Ultrasound

2.2.1 Introduction

Facial ultrasound has become an invaluable tool in the field of aesthetic medicine, providing clinicians with real-time, non-invasive imaging capabilities for precise anatomical assessments. The quality of ultrasound images is paramount for accurate diagnosis and effective procedural planning. This section explores the scientific principles and advancements in image optimization techniques specifically tailored for facial ultrasound.

The choice of transducer and its frequency significantly influence image quality. In facial ultrasound, where fine structures and superficial tissues are of interest, high-frequency transducers (e.g., 10–15 MHz) are preferred. These transducers offer enhanced resolution, enabling the visualization of subtle facial features and superficial vascular structures. Careful consideration of the depth of penetration versus resolution is crucial in selecting the optimal transducer frequency for different facial regions.

Optimal probe positioning and angulation play a pivotal role in maximizing image clarity. Proper contact with the skin surface, ensuring perpendicular alignment, and maintaining a consistent gel interface are essential for reducing artifacts and obtaining accurate representations of facial structures. Clinicians must be attentive to the patient's comfort during the ultrasound procedure, as optimal probe positioning may vary based on the specific facial area under examination. Fine-tuning gain settings is a critical aspect of image optimization. Adjusting gain controls allows for the optimization of image brightness and contrast, ensuring that subtle tissue variations are adequately visualized. Furthermore, careful management of the dynamic range is essential to capture a wide spectrum of echogenicity within the facial tissues. Balancing these parameters enhances the overall visibility of anatomical details and facilitates a more accurate interpretation of ultrasound images [9].

Advanced image optimization techniques include frequency compounding and harmonic imaging. Frequency compounding involves combining data obtained at different frequencies to improve image quality and reduce noise, particularly in superficial tissues. Harmonic imaging utilizes the harmonic frequencies generated by tissues, which can enhance resolution and contrast while minimizing artifacts. These techniques are particularly beneficial when visualizing facial structures with varying acoustic properties.

2.2.2 Knobology During Sonographic Imaging in Facial Aesthetics

The process of image optimization in medical ultrasound is governed by a variety of settings collectively known as ultrasound knobology. While key components and functionalities are maintained across ultrasound systems produced by different manufacturers, variations in layout may exist among vendors.

Among the considerations in ultrasound system operation is the selection of the imaging mode, a pivotal determinant of diagnostic output. Predominantly, the Brightness mode (B-mode) stands out as the most frequently employed modality for standard grayscale imaging. For the assessment of vascular flow, the Color mode (C-mode) is utilized, whereas the Power mode (P-mode) is instrumental in evaluating energy. Additionally, Pulsed Wave spectral tracing (PW mode) is indispensable for certain diagnostic applications to assess arterial occlusion by means of thorough assessment of vascular flow rates.

Critical to the optimization process is the manipulation of various parameters. Gain adjustment plays a pivotal role in controlling the overall brightness of the image, contributing significantly to contrast enhancement. Focus, another parameter, influences the depth and clarity of the imaged structures, adding an element of precision to the diagnostic process.

Furthermore, Tissue Gain Compensation (TGC) is an essential component in the optimization toolkit, serving to rectify variations in tissue echogenicity at different depths, thereby ensuring uniform image quality throughout the examination. This parameter is particularly pertinent in mitigating the impact of tissue attenuation (define tissue attenuation).

In the realm of workflow optimization, the establishment of presets tailored to frequent areas of interest within a clinician's practice is imperative. Collaborative efforts with a vendor's application specialist or an on-site sonographic expert are integral to the development of such presets, fostering a standardized approach during patient assessments. These presets should not only encompass topographic maps detailing the location of the ultrasound examination but also feature toggle indicators that elucidate the orientation of the transducer during imaging. Such meticulous documentation ensures reproducibility, enabling consistent and reliable imaging across multiple sessions.

A comprehensive understanding and proficient manipulation of ultrasound knobology, encompassing imaging modes and parameter adjustments, coupled with the implementation of tailored presets, are indispensable for achieving optimal image quality and workflow efficiency in clinical ultrasound applications.

Figure 2.7 allows a representation of these settings.

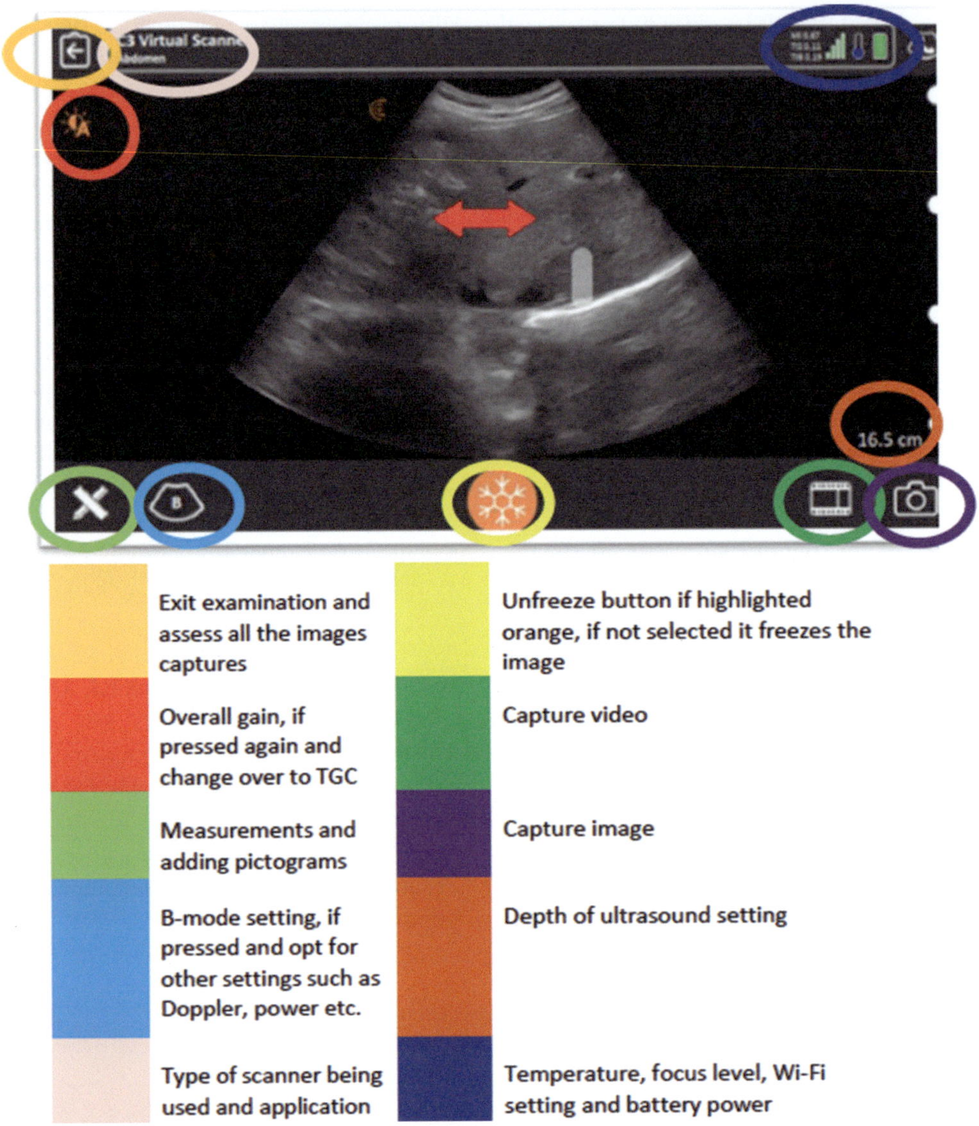

Fig. 2.7 Ultrasound knobology
Various ultrasound manufacturers boast various knobology interfaces, however the principles remain similar across various units. In this image, the layout of the Clarius HD3 system is demonstrated as part of a point of care ultrasound system

2.3 Colour and Power Doppler Technique in Facial Aesthetics

2.3.1 Introduction

Facial aesthetics involves the comprehensive assessment and enhancement of facial features to achieve a harmonious and pleasing appearance. In recent years, diagnostic imaging techniques have played a crucial role in understanding facial anatomy and optimizing safety with aesthetic procedures. Among these techniques, Color Doppler and Power Doppler imaging have emerged as valuable tools, providing insights into vascular dynamics and aiding practitioners in planning and executing facial aesthetic interventions. Color Doppler imaging is a non-invasive ultrasound-based technique that visualizes blood flow within vessels. In facial aesthetics, this technique can be applied to assess the vascularity of various facial structures, including skin, subcutaneous tissues, and muscles. By using the color flow pattern representations during imaging, practitioners can identify blood flow patterns (red blood flow indicates motion towards the transducer and blue color refers to blood moving away from transducer), detect abnormalities, and evaluate the perfusion of tissues. This information is crucial in preoperative planning for procedures such as dermal fillers, botulinum toxin injections, and facelifts, where an understanding of vascular supply helps mitigate the risk of complications. Power Doppler imaging, an extension of Color Doppler, provides additional advantages in assessing low-velocity blood flow that is not reliant on the direction of blood flow. This technique is particularly beneficial in visualizing microvascular structures, making it relevant in facial aesthetic procedures that involve delicate and intricate vascular networks. Power Doppler can enhance the detection of subtle changes in blood flow, aiding practitioners in avoiding potential complications related to vascular compromise during aesthetic interventions [5, 14–16].

Color and Power Doppler techniques enable practitioners to map the vascular anatomy of the face accurately. This information is vital for avoiding inadvertent injection into vessels during procedures like dermal filler placements, minimizing the risk of vascular occlusion and associated complications. Real-time visualization of blood flow with Doppler techniques aids in immediate recognition of vascular compromise during procedures. This allows for prompt intervention to minimize potential complications, such as ischemia or necrosis [5, 14–16].

The integration of Color and Power Doppler techniques into facial aesthetic practices provides a valuable dimension to preoperative planning and intraoperative monitoring. These techniques contribute to enhanced safety and precision in various aesthetic procedures, ensuring optimal outcomes and patient satisfaction. As technology continues to advance, the role of Doppler imaging in facial aesthetics is likely to expand, further refining the practice of aesthetic medicine.

2.3.2 Practical Application of Color Doppler in Facial Aesthetics

The various modes of ultrasound provide varying qualitative and quantitative output on the resulting sonographic image. B mode provides a grayscale image, based on the amplitude of the receiving sonographic signal. Color Doppler provides a blue/red color image based on the velocity of moving objects through use of a sample volume over an area of interest.

Power Doppler provides an orange/red color image based on the energy of the returning Doppler signal, as opposed to the frequency of the B-mode imaging output. Power Doppler recognizes multiple shift frequencies due to flow and develops a range of echoes, in the form of an orange/red color map.

The subsequent frequency produced is not included in the resultant Power Doppler image, rather the amplitude of the incoming signal is used for the resultant image. The advantage of using Power Doppler for aesthetic imaging is that it is not dependent on the Doppler angle and can recognize vascular flow near the ultrasound beam.

Various image optimization techniques should be considered upon use of color Doppler for patient assessment [5, 11, 14].

2.3.2.1 Color Gain

The use of color gain produces an increase in the amplitude of returning signal to the probe. The purpose of its use is to enhance the visibility of color flow in the region of interest. It is important to note, as with B-mode gain, increasing the color gain too much would lead to over amplification of the returning signal, producing flow presence in non-vascular regions. On the same note, decreasing the color gain too much, would lead to lack of presence of flow in a region of interest. The best practice for its use, is to incrementally increase the Color gain (Fig. 2.8), until blooming appears, and to then reduce the gain slightly for optimal image output [5, 14–16].

2.3.2.2 Pulse Repetition Frequency

Adjusting the PRF scale (Fig. 2.9), changes the number of pulses per second emitted from the

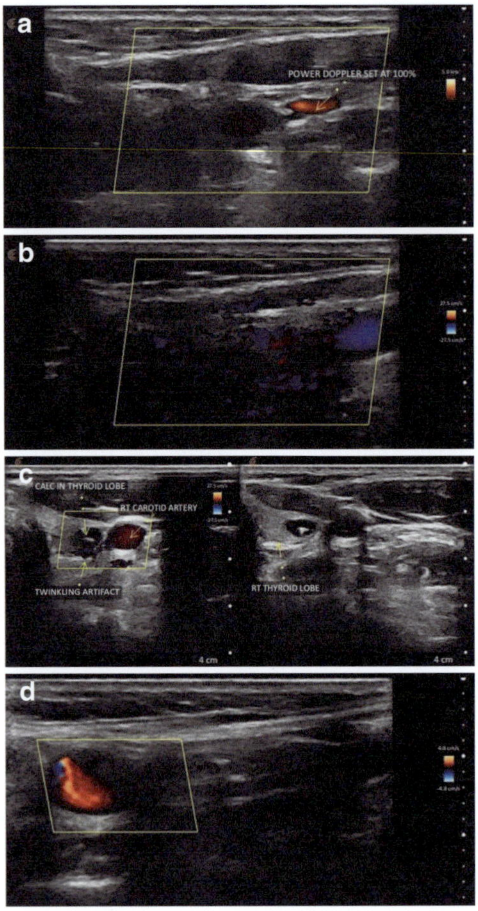

Fig. 2.8 (**a**–**d**) Color gain. (**a**) Blooming or color bleed artifact occurs when the color signal indicating blood flow extends beyond its true boundaries, spreading into adjacent regions with no actual flow. (**b**) The image sequence shows the right carotid artery inlongitudinal orientation, whilst the colour gain is gradually increased. The causing factor is the colour-write priority which represents a threshold above which no B-mode (grayscale) pixels can be overwritten by colour signal. (**c**) Twinkling artifact. It occurs as a focus of alternating colors on Doppler signal behind a reflective object which gives the appearance of turbulent blood flow. The underlying mechanism of this artifact is thought to be a result of inherent noise within the ultrasound scanner, specifically phase (a.k.a. clock) jitter within the Doppler electronics. In this image a calcification within a colloid cyst of the right thyroid lobe produces the so-called twinkling artifact, adjacent to the right carotid artery in transverse plane. (**d**) Common Carotid Artery (CCA) scanned with an inappropriately low PRF (1.4 kHz) for the high velocity arterial flow. As a result flow above the upper threshold of is displayed with blue hues, during the systolic peak

probe. If the PRF is set high, it can demonstrate higher scale velocities as for example in arteries. If the PRF is set too low, it will be able to demonstrate low scale velocities as can be seen in veins. If the PRF is set too high, it would lead to aliasing, where the range of frequencies are beyond the Doppler range, thus leading to loss of directional and velocity information. Aliasing can be useful in detecting areas of vessel stenosis [15].

2.3.2.3 Sample Volume Size

Setting a sample volume box (Fig. 2.10), allows interrogation of a specific anatomical region of interest. If the sample volume is set too large, it would lead to oversampling and loss of temporal resolution/frame rate. For PW doppler, the sample box should be set as 2/3 of the target vessel's entire lumen diameter [5, 14–16].

2.3.2.4 Doppler Angle

It is important to adjust the Doppler angle of incident (Figure 2.11) sound waves to optimize flow information. The Doppler angle refers to the angle created between the axis of the ultrasound beam and the direction of blood flow in a vessel (refer to Fig. 2.11). To detect flow efficiently an optimal angle is required. The optimal angle is set at 60°; however, less than 60° is also considered acceptable as small variations in the optimal angle produces minimal changes to the resultant calculated velocity [5, 14–16].

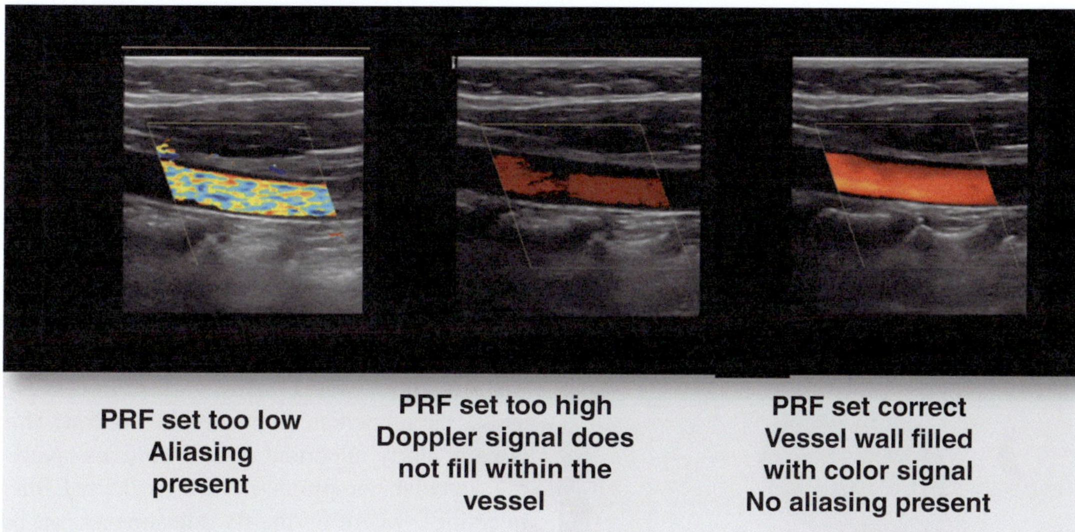

Fig. 2.9 Pulse Repetition Frequency (PRF) scale depicts the variance in imaging when the PRF setting is set too low or high in comparison to correct PRF setting when no aliasing is present

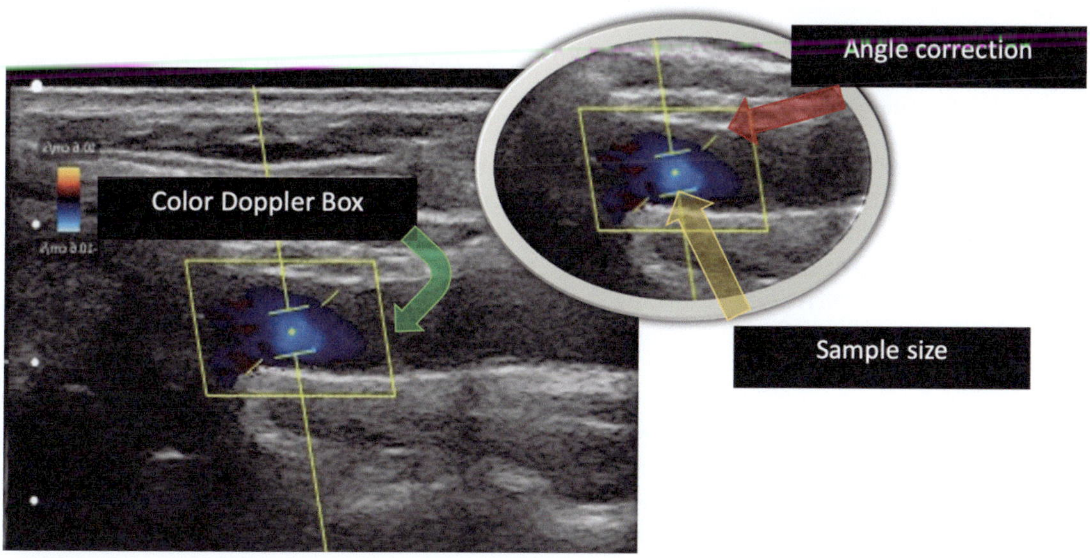

Fig. 2.10 Sample volume size
The use of the color box during Spectral Doppler imaging demonstrates the use of angle correction and the sample size (red arrows). This function can be altered according to the artery being assessed for angle and size/caliber of the vessel

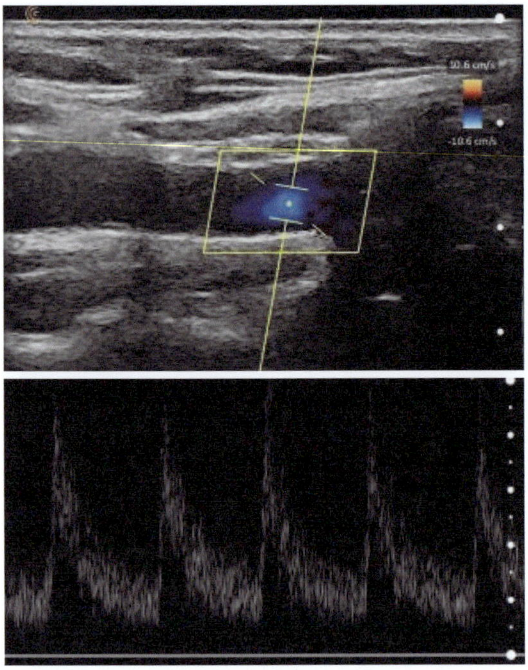

Fig. 2.11 Doppler angle
Doppler angle is used at a 60° angle or less to ensure optimal doppler shift frequency is obtained during Spectral imaging
Note the use of the angle correction and sample size for specific artery caliber

2.4 Spectral Doppler Techniques in Facial Aesthetics

2.4.1 Introduction

Spectral Doppler relies on the Doppler effect, where the frequency shift of reflected ultrasound waves from moving blood cells is analyzed to determine the velocity and direction of blood flow. In facial aesthetics, this technique allows for the quantification of blood flow characteristics, including peak systolic velocity, end-diastolic velocity, and resistive index. By understanding these parameters, practitioners can gain insights into the vascular health of facial tissues and make informed decisions during aesthetic procedures [16].

Spectral Doppler techniques enable a detailed evaluation of the blood vessels supplying facial structures. This information is crucial in preoperative planning for procedures such as vascularized tissue transfers, where knowledge of vessel caliber and flow characteristics is essential for successful outcomes.

Aesthetic interventions, such as facelifts and liposuction, can impact the hemodynamics of facial blood vessels. Spectral Doppler provides a means to assess changes in blood flow patterns, helping practitioners anticipate and mitigate potential complications related to altered vascular dynamics.

Real-time Spectral Doppler monitoring during aesthetic procedures allows practitioners to assess the immediate impact on blood flow. This is particularly important in interventions involving vascular compromise, such as dermal filler injections, where on-the-fly adjustments can be made to enhance patient safety.

Spectral Doppler imaging aids in postoperative evaluation by assessing the effects of interventions on blood flow. This contributes to the long-term success of procedures, especially in cases involving tissue flaps, fat grafts, or other vascularized grafts. There are two subsets of Spectral Doppler, namely Pulsed Wave and Continuous Wave Spectral Doppler [16].

A prospective trajectory in the field involves the incorporation of three-dimensional (3D) Spectral Doppler imaging. This approach holds promise for offering a more comprehensive understanding of the intricate three-dimensional vascular architecture of the face, thereby enabling practitioners to plan and execute aesthetic interventions with unparalleled accuracy. Concurrently, advancements in quantitative hemodynamic analysis aim to provide more precise measurements of blood flow parameters. Enhanced algorithms and software tools may facilitate automated analysis, mitigating subjectivity in interpretations and augmenting the reproducibility of results in clinical practice.

Integration with artificial intelligence (AI) represents another frontier of exploration. AI algorithms may contribute to real-time analysis, automating the detection of subtle changes in blood flow patterns and furnishing immediate feedback to practitioners during procedures. This integration holds potential to enhance efficiency, accuracy, and safety in facial aesthetic interventions. Furthermore, ongoing efforts in the miniaturization of Spectral Doppler devices and the development of portable, point-of-care solutions are noteworthy. Such advancements could broaden the accessibility of vascular assessments, allowing for their incorporation into diverse clinical settings, including outpatient clinics and aesthetic practice offices [17].

The synergy of Spectral Doppler with other functional imaging modalities, such as contrast-enhanced ultrasound and elastography, is also under investigation. This combined approach could furnish a more holistic assessment of tissue perfusion and elasticity, aiding practitioners in tailoring interventions to individual patient characteristics. Additionally, the prospect of correlating Spectral Doppler findings with clinical outcomes is an area of interest. Establishing predictive models based on preoperative vascular assessments may empower practitioners to anticipate challenges and customize treatment plans for optimal results, thereby further improving patient safety and satisfaction. Beyond the confines of facial aesthetics, the research horizon envisions the exploration of Spectral Doppler's utility in assessing dermatological conditions, wound healing, and other therapeutic interventions. As these scientific inquiries progress, the integration of these advancements into clinical practice holds the potential to redefine the landscape of aesthetic medicine, ushering in a new era characterized by heightened precision, safety, and patient-centric outcomes [17].

2.4.2 Spectral Waveform Analysis in Facial Aesthetics

The standard spectral pulse wave Doppler tracing (Fig. 2.12) contains both a clear spectral window as well as a strong systole/diastole flow rate upon imaging. Spectral window refers to the area underneath the wave pattern seen on ultrasound, appearing "clear", without filling underneath the tracing line. This is demonstrated with below figures as a method of determining vascular impedance when the spectral window does not appear "clear" [16].

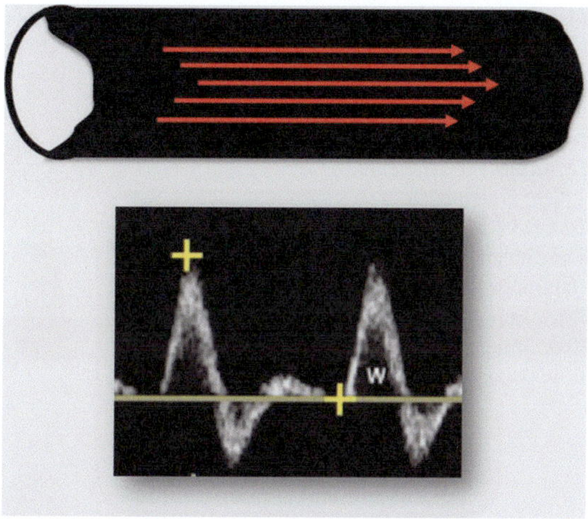

Fig. 2.12 Normal Spectral Pulse Wave tracing
This image demonstrates a clear spectral window with no signs of arterial flow being imposed by any intra-arterial occlusion
This image demonstrates normal laminar flow, with the majority of red blood cells moving within the vessel lumen in the same direction without any occlusion/obstruction of flow

The frequency spectrum shows blood flow relative to the transducer. Flow in one direction, toward the transducer, is displayed above the spectrum baseline, and flow in the opposite direction is shown below the baseline.

2.4.3 Acceleration and Pulsatility Index

With regards to pulsatility index, in arteries, each cycle of cardiac activity produces a distinct wave on the Doppler frequency spectrum that begins with systole and terminates at the end of diastole. The term waveform refers to the shape of each of these waves, and this shape, in turn, defines a very important flow property called pulsatility. In general terms, Doppler waveforms have low, moderate, or high pulsatility features, depending on the region where the artery resides and the size of the lumen, which affects the rate of pulsatility within a vessel.

Figure 2.13 demonstrates the three most common pulsatility wave forms as either, high, moderate, or low.

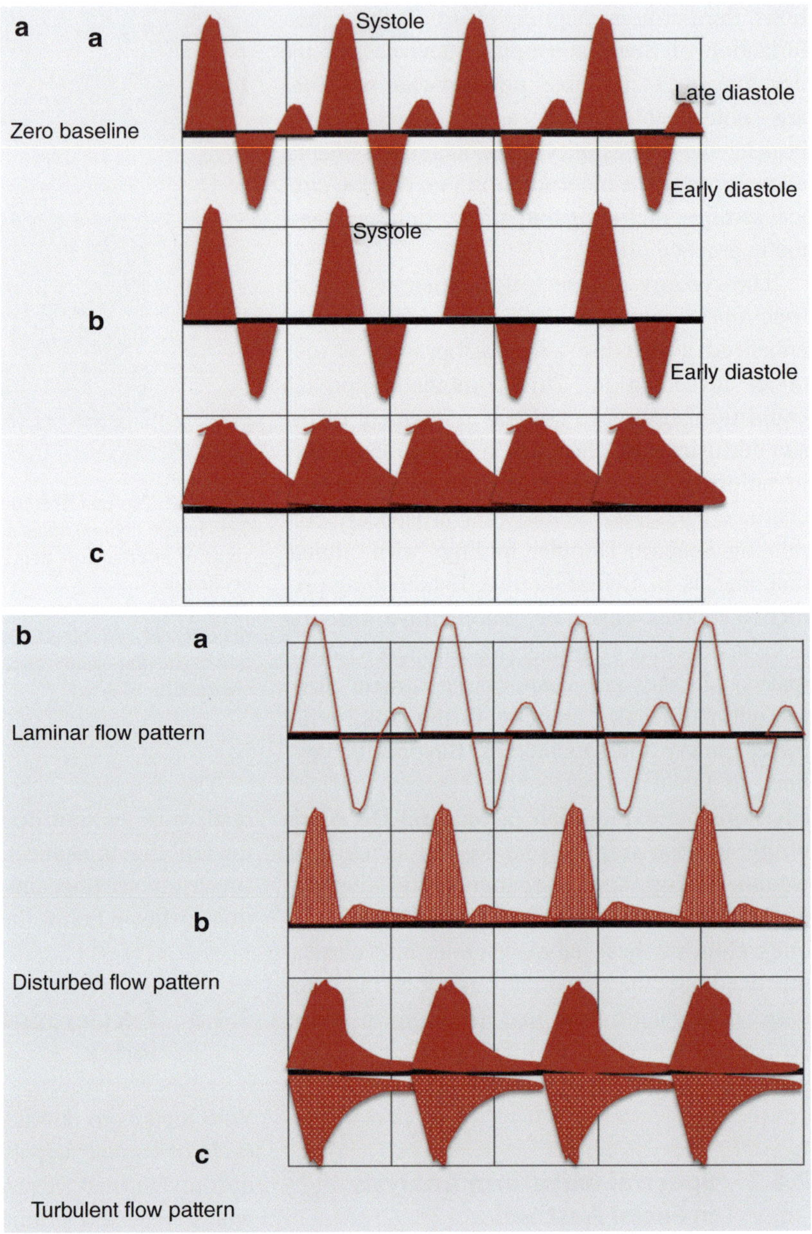

Fig. 2.13 (**a**) Pulsatility index of arteries. (**b**) Disturbed flow patterns related to arterial occlusion
(**a**) Image A: Triphasic. Image B: Biphasic. Image C: Monophasic waveforms
(**b**) Image A: Laminar flow. Image B: disturbed flow. Image C: Turbulent flow patterns

(A) Low pulsatility is indicated by broad systolic peaks and persistent forward flow throughout the diastole (e.g., the internal carotid artery).
(B) Moderate pulsatility is indicated by tall, sharp, narrow systolic peaks and relatively little diastolic flow (e.g., the external carotid artery).
(C) High pulsatility is characterized by narrow systolic peaks, flow reversal early in diastole, and absence of flow late in diastole.

In this classic triphasic example, the first phase (1) is systole, the second phase (2) is brief diastolic flow reversal, and the third phase (3) is diastolic forward flow. Triphasic flow is seen in normal extremity arteries at rest [16].

Acceleration is another important flow feature evident in Doppler spectral waveforms. In most normal situations, red cells in an artery accelerate very rapidly during systole, and the peak velocity

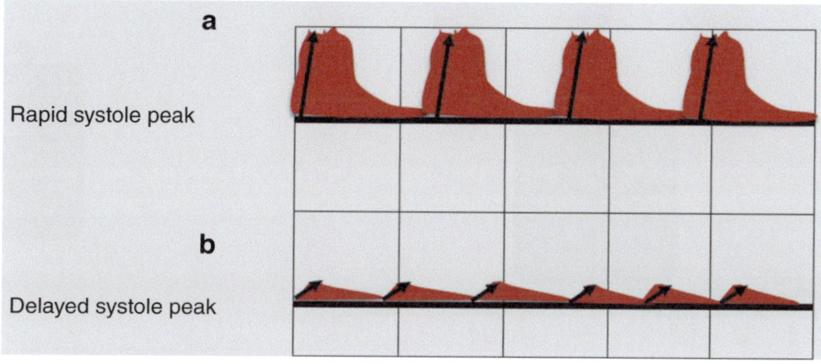

Fig. 2.14 Acceleration differences during arterial occlusion Image A: Rapid systole peak at 90° Image B: delayed systole peak not at 90° demonstrating signs of damping/arterial occlusion

is reached within a few hundredths of a second after ventricular contraction begins. Rapid acceleration produces an almost vertical deflection of the Doppler waveform at the start of the systole.

In Fig. 2.14, the difference between a normal rapid systolic and a delayed ventricular contraction and systolic upstroke on the Spectral trace waveform is demonstrated [16].

The above analysis methods are considered advanced techniques in assessing the presence of an arterial occlusion during filler injection or for other facial reconstructive surgery performed. If the use of Spectral pulse wave is promoted daily, it may promote confidence, and be considered a valued tool for arterial assessment pre and post during facial aesthetic treatments.

2.5 Common Pitfalls During Facial Ultrasound

2.5.1 Artifact Analysis During Sonographic Imaging

Artifacts can impede accurate interpretation of ultrasound images. Awareness of common artifacts such as acoustic shadowing, reverberation, and side lobes is crucial. Implementation of techniques such as tissue harmonic imaging, spatial compounding, and beam steering can mitigate artifacts and improve image quality. Continuous education and training for clinicians in artifact recognition and reduction contribute to the proficiency of facial ultrasound examinations [1–6].

Ultrasound artifacts (Fig. 2.15) are inherent to the imaging process and can influence the accuracy and interpretation of ultrasound images. Clinicians need to be well-versed in recognizing and mitigating these artifacts for precise diagnostic assessments. Here, we elaborate on some common types of ultrasound artifacts:

Acoustic shadowing occurs when the ultrasound beam encounters a highly reflective or attenuating structure, causing a shadow to be cast beyond the structure. This artifact can obscure details in the deeper tissues, limiting the visualization of structures lying behind highly reflective interfaces. Adjusting the angle of incidence or utilizing alternate imaging planes can help minimize the impact of acoustic shadowing.

Reverberation artifacts result from the bouncing of ultrasound waves between two strong reflectors, creating multiple, parallel echoes on the display. This gives the appearance of evenly spaced lines that may obscure underlying structures. Techniques such as adjusting the gain settings or altering the angle of incidence can help reduce reverberation artifacts.

Mirror image artifacts occur when the ultrasound beam reflects off a strong reflector and returns to the transducer, creating a false image on the opposite side of the true structure. This can lead to misinterpretation of anatomical features. Adjusting the angle of incidence and using additional imaging planes can help differentiate between the true and mirror images.

Edge shadowing results from the refraction of ultrasound waves at tissue interfaces, causing a hypoechoic shadow to appear distal to the edge of a structure. This artifact can affect the

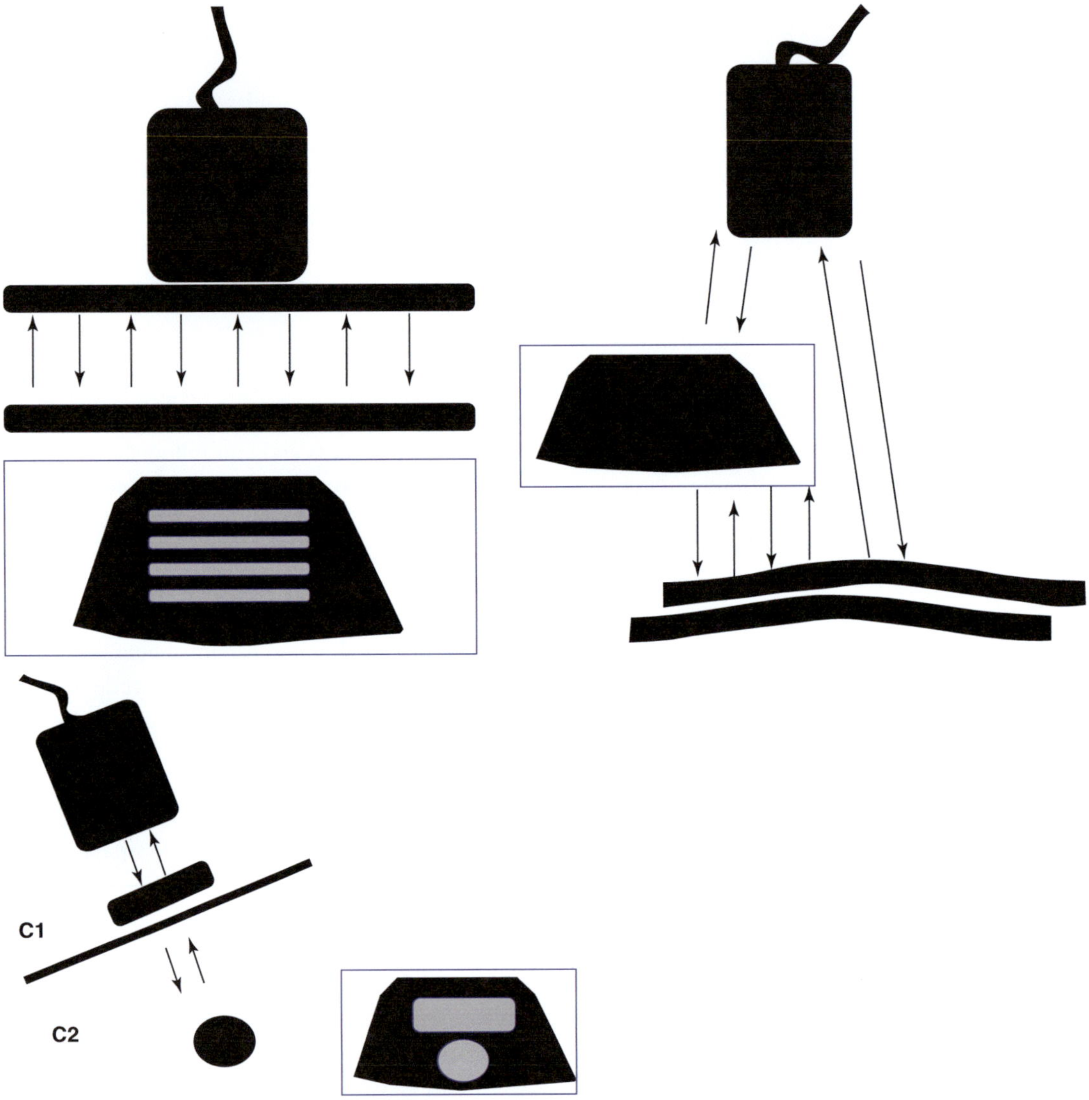

Fig. 2.15 Artifacts in B mode ultrasound imaging
Image 1: Reverberation artifact
Diagram shows ultrasound echoes being repeatedly reflected between two highly reflective interfaces. The display shows multiple equally spaced signals extending into the deep field
Image 2: Mirror image artifact
In this diagram, the gray arrows represent the expected reflective path of the ultrasound beam. These echoes are displayed properly. The black arrows show an alternative path of the primary ultrasound beam. In this path, the primary ultrasound beam encounters the deeper reflective interface first. The echoes from the deeper reflective interface take longer to return to the transducer and are misplaced on the display
Image 3: Refraction artifact
Diagram shows the refraction or change in direction of the obliquely angled incident ultrasound beam as it travels between two adjacent tissues with different sound propagation velocities (C1 and C2). The incident ultrasound beam with refraction encounters two structures. The object in the path of the refracted portion of the beam is misplaced because the processor assumes a straight path of the beam

delineation of boundaries and should be considered when interpreting images. Adjusting the gain settings and using imaging techniques that reduce edge artifacts can improve overall image quality.

Lobe artifacts occur when ultrasound beams deviate from the main beam direction, generating additional weaker lobes. These secondary lobes can produce false echoes, leading to the misrepresentation of structures. Beam steering and focusing techniques are employed to minimize lobe artifacts and enhance the accuracy of ultrasound images.

Clutter artifacts manifest as low-level echoes spread across the image, often obscuring subtle details. These artifacts can be caused by the presence of scattered echoes from structures outside the main imaging plane. Adjusting the gain and filtering settings can help reduce clutter artifacts and improve the overall clarity of the ultrasound image.

Comet tail artifacts, also known as comet tail reverberation, appear as a dense, comet-like tail trailing a strong reflector. These artifacts can create false echoes and impact the visualization of structures. (Fig. 2.16) Modifying the gain and time-gain compensation settings can help mitigate comet tail artifacts, allowing for a more accurate representation of the underlying anatomy [6].

Understanding these common ultrasound artifacts is essential for clinicians to optimize image quality and make accurate diagnostic interpretations. Ongoing education and training in artifact recognition and mitigation strategies contribute to the proficiency of ultrasound practitioners in various medical specialties, including aesthetic medicine.

Optimizing facial ultrasound images involves a multifaceted approach, encompassing transducer selection, probe positioning, gain adjustment, advanced imaging techniques, and artifact reduction. As technology continues to advance, the integration of novel technologies and continuous refinement of imaging protocols will further elevate the role of facial ultrasound in aesthetic medicine, enabling clinicians to make informed decisions and enhance patient outcomes.

2.5.2 Sonographic Appearance of Fillers on Ultrasound Images

The sonographic appearance of various fillers used in facial aesthetics is a critical aspect of preoperative planning and postoperative assessment, providing clinicians with valuable insights into the distribution, characteristics, and potential complications associated with these substances. Different fillers exhibit distinct sonographic features based on their composition, density, and interaction with ultrasound waves. Here, we explore the sonographic appearance in echogenicity of common fillers used in facial aesthetics [7, 8, 10–13, 18, 19]:

Hyaluronic acid (HA) fillers, being a natural component of the extracellular matrix, generally exhibit low echogenicity on ultrasound imaging. They appear as hypoechoic or anechoic regions, blending with the surrounding tissues. The homogeneous and low-density appearance of HA fillers facilitates differentiation from adjacent anatomical structures. In cases of vascular compromise, HA fillers may exhibit increased echogenicity due to edema or inflammation. Examples of HA fillers include: Juvéderm (e.g., Juvéderm Ultra, Juvéderm Voluma), Restylane (e.g., Restylane-L, Restylane Lyft), Belotero (e.g., Belotero Balance) [7, 8, 10–13, 18, 19]

Calcium Hydroxyapatite (CaHa) fillers, composed of microspheres suspended in a gel carrier, typically display moderate to high echogenicity on ultrasound. This increased echogenicity is attributed to the calcium microspheres, which reflect ultrasound waves effectively. The sonographic appearance of CaHA fillers is often described as hyperechoic or bright echoes within the soft tissue, allowing for clear delineation during imaging. Examples of CaHA fillers include Radiesse and Harmonica [7, 8, 10–13, 18, 19].

Poly-L-Lactic Acid (PLLA) Fillers designed to stimulate collagen production, may initially appear hyperechoic due to the microsphere component. However, over time, as collagen synthesis is induced, the echogenicity may decrease, resulting in a more homogeneous and hypoechoic appearance. This evolving sonographic pattern

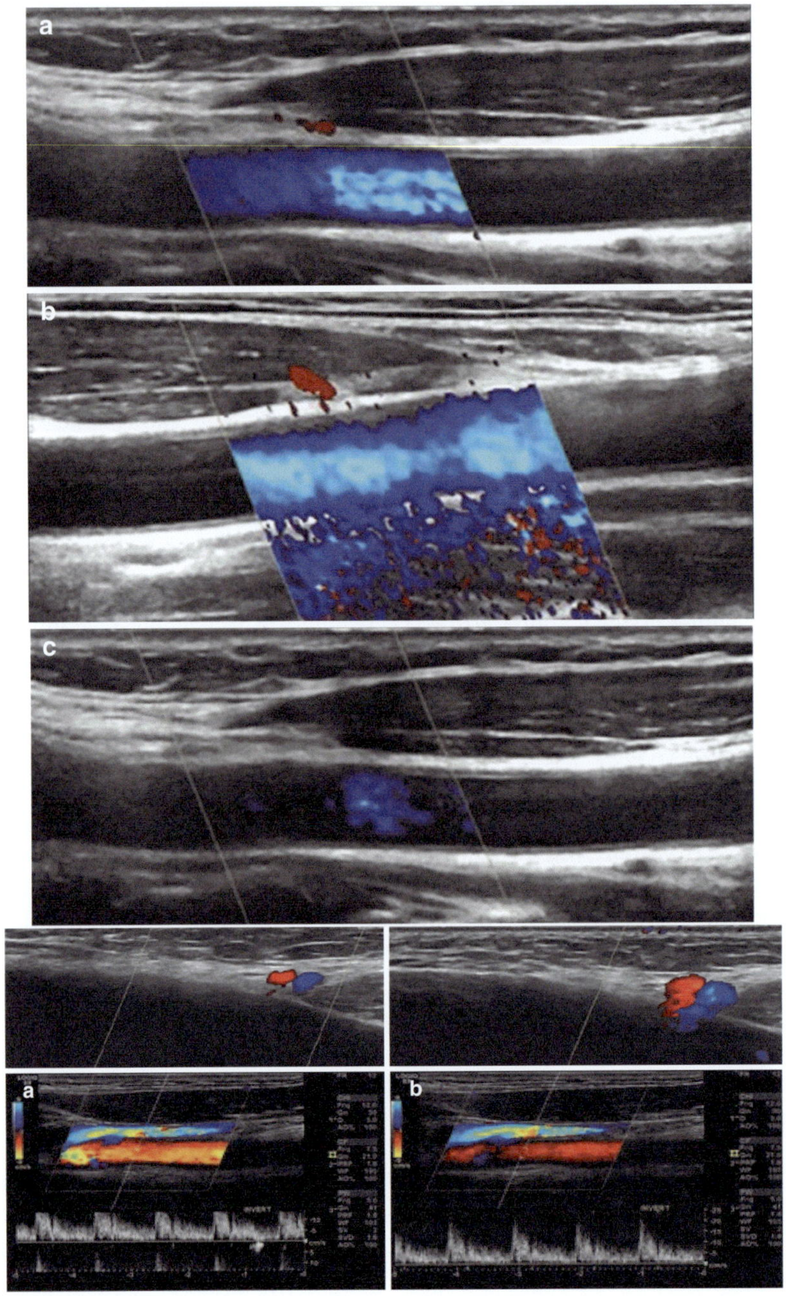

Fig. 2.16 Ultrasound artifacts in color doppler imaging
Image 1: Color gain variances
(**a**) Top image Colour gain just right
(**b**) Middle image. Color gain too high
(**c**) Bottom image. Color gain too low
Image 2: Blooming in facial artery
Left image indicates correct usage of color gain for the facial artery, just anterior to the masseter muscle
Right image indicates color gain set too high, causing blooming of facial artery
Image 3: Baseline correction in spectral doppler. (**a**) left image refers to incorrect placement of baseline (**b**) refers to moving of baseline level so that the systole flow can be visualised

reflects the dynamic nature of PLLA fillers in promoting tissue regeneration. Example includes Sculptra [7, 8, 10–13, 18, 19].

Polymethyl Methacrylate (PMMA) Fillers, comprising microspheres in a collagen carrier, typically present as hyperechoic structures on ultrasound. The presence of microspheres contributes to their increased echogenicity. PMMA fillers may also exhibit posterior shadowing, a characteristic artifact that can impact the visualization of structures behind the filler material. Example of PMMA include Bellafill [7, 8, 10–13, 18, 19].

Autologous fat grafts, obtained through liposuction and subsequently injected, can vary in echogenicity based on factors such as processing techniques and the presence of oil or blood components. Fat grafts often appear hypoechoic initially, resembling the surrounding adipose tissue. Over time, fat grafts may undergo changes, and echogenicity may increase due to fibrous tissue formation or cystic degeneration.

Collagen fillers, though less commonly used in recent years, can be visualized on ultrasound as hypoechoic structures. The echogenicity may vary based on the collagen concentration and the presence of additives (Fig. 2.17). Collagen fillers are often distinguishable from surrounding tissues due to their unique sonographic characteristics. Examples of temporary fillers include Cosmoderm and Zyderm [10, 13, 19].

Incorporating color Doppler and power Doppler imaging in facial ultrasound provides valuable information about blood flow dynamics. Optimization of Doppler settings involves adjusting scale, pulse repetition frequency, and wall filter to enhance sensitivity and reduce aliasing artifacts. Careful consideration of these settings allows for accurate assessment of vascularity in facial tissues, aiding in preoperative planning and the avoidance of vascular complications during aesthetic procedures.

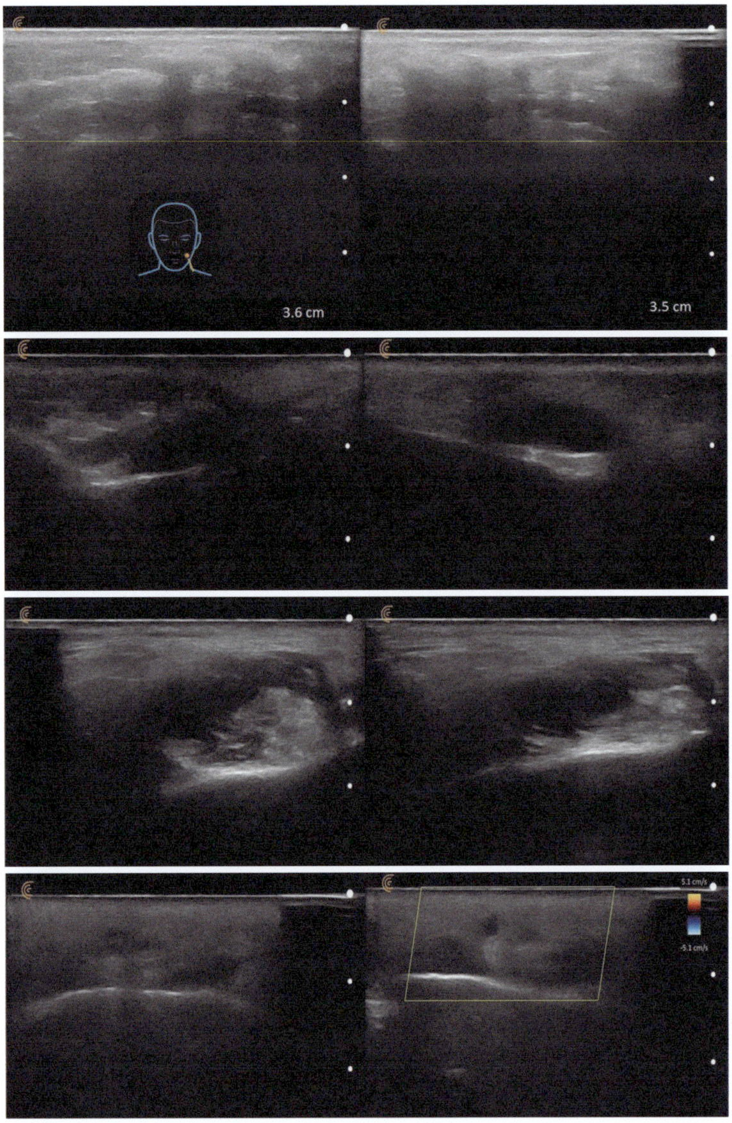

Fig. 2.17 Pictorial review of various fillers as demonstrated with ultrasound imaging
Example 1: Main filler ingredient is Synthetic calcium hydroxyapatite
Note the casting posterior acoustic shadowing due to calcium deposits within the filler content. The filler was placed in the subcutaneous soft tissue of the masseter region 4/12 ago. Probe is in a transverse oblique plane, across the left masseter muscle belly
Example 2: Main ingredient is crosslinked hyaluronic acid (HA)
Recently placed HA filler has a similar appearance to a simple cyst, with clear hypoechoic contents and well circumscribed oval border. The probe is in a longitudinal plane, just lateral to the nasolabial fold within the piriform recess, image split to demonstrate bilateral recess
Example 3: Main ingredient is crosslinked hyaluronic acid (HA)
This example demonstrated degrading and integration of filler product into surrounding soft tissue, in comparison to Example 2, the fluid contents, now appears complex with mixed echogenic internal foci present. The probe is in a transverse plane, across the masseter muscle, with filler placed within the superficial muscle bellyExample 4: Main ingredient is synthetic calcium hydroxyapatite in the mentum regionDegrading and integration of old filler is noted with small microcalcifications noted within the fluid bolus, 3/12 of age. Noted posterior acoustic casting shadow due to calcific contents of the filler product

References

1. Wu WT, Chang KV, Chang HC, Chen LR, Kuan CH, Kao JT, et al. Ultrasound imaging of the facial muscles and relevance with Botulinum toxin injections: a pictorial essay and narrative review. Toxins (Basel). 2022;14(2) https://doi.org/10.3390/toxins14020101.
2. Zetlaoui PJ, Gauthier E, Benhamou D. Ultrasound-guided scalp nerve blocks for neurosurgery: a narrative review. Anaesth Crit Care Pain Med. 2020;39(6):876–82. https://doi.org/10.1016/j.accpm.2020.06.019.
3. Bhoi S, Chandra A, Galwankar S. Ultrasound-guided nerve blocks in the emergency department. J Emerg Trauma Shock. 2010;3(1):82–8. https://doi.org/10.4103/0974-2700.58655.
4. Ryu JH, Shim JH, Yeom JH, Shin WJ, Cho SY, Jeon WJ. Ultrasound-guided greater occipital nerve block with botulinum toxin for patients with chronic headache in the occipital area: a randomized controlled trial. Korean J Anesthesiol. 2019;72(5):479–85. https://doi.org/10.4097/kja.19145.
5. Kim SH. Interpretation of peripheral arterial and venous Doppler waveforms: a consensus statement from the Society for Vascular Medicine and Society for vascular ultrasound. Vasc Med. 2020;25(5):484–506.
6. Gerr A [Internet]. Anisotropy as most important pitfall in ultrasound imaging. 2023. Available from: www.sonoskills.com.
7. Sundaram H, Signorini M, Liew S, Trindade de Almeida AR, Wu Y, Vieira Braz A, et al. Global Aesthetics Consensus: Botulinum Toxin Type A--Evidence-Based Review, Emerging Concepts, and Consensus Recommendations for Aesthetic Use, Including Updates on Complications. Plast Reconstr Surg 2016; 137(3):518e-529e. https://doi.org/10.1097/01.prs.0000475758.63709.23.
8. Samizadeh S, De Boulle K. Complications of toxins and fillers in facial aesthetics. Prim Dent J. 2023;12(3):65–72.
9. Malherbe K. Image-guided injection techniques. Pretoria: Boutique Book Publishers; 2023.
10. Beer K. Dermal fillers and combinations of fillers for facial rejuvenation. Dermatol Clin. 2009;27(4):427–32. https://doi.org/10.1016/j.det.2009.08.011.
11. Rayess HM, Svider PF, Hanba C, Patel VS, DeJoseph LM, Carron M, et al. A cross-sectional analysis of adverse events and litigation for injectable fillers. JAMA Facial Plast Surg. 2018;20(3):207–14. https://doi.org/10.1001/jamafacial.2017.1888.
12. Daines SM, Williams EF. Complications associated with injectable soft-tissue fillers: a 5-year retrospective review. JAMA Facial Plast Surg. 2013;15(3):226–31. https://doi.org/10.1001/jamafacial.2013.798.
13. Arlette JP, Trotter MJ. Anatomic location of hyaluronic acid filler material injected into nasolabial fold: a histologic study. Dermatologic Surg. 2008;34(Suppl 1):S56–62. https://doi.org/10.1111/j.1524-4725.2008.34244.x. discussion S-3
14. Tucunduva MJ, Tucunduva-Neto R, Saieg M, Costa AL, de Freitas C. Vascular mapping of the face: B-mode and doppler ultrasonography study. Med Oral Patol Oral Cir Bucal. 2016;21(2):e135–41. https://doi.org/10.4317/medoral.20754.
15. Shah A, Irshad A. Sonography doppler flow imaging instrumentation. Statpearls; 2024.
16. Key R [Internet]. Doppler Flow Imaging and Spectral Analysis 2017 [5 September 2022]. Available from: https://www.radiologykey.com/spectralanalysis.
17. Ambroziak M, Noszczyk B, Pietruski P, Guz W, Paluch L. Elastography reference values of facial skin elasticity. Postepy Dermatol Alergol. 2019;36(5):626–34. https://doi.org/10.5114/ada.2018.77502.
18. Papageorgiou K, Chang HS, Isaacs D, Fiaschetti D, Ang M, Goldberg R. Refining the goals of oculofacial rejuvenation with dynamic ultrasonography. Aesthet Surg J. 2012;32(2):207–19. https://doi.org/10.1177/1090820X11434523.
19. Alam M, Dover JS. Management of complications and sequelae with temporary injectable fillers. Plast Reconstr Surg. 2007;120(6 Suppl):98S–105S. https://doi.org/10.1097/01.prs.0000248859.14788.60.

3 Anatomical Principles of the Face

The surface anatomy of the face (Fig. 3.1) and its correlated use with ultrasound is important during aesthetic imaging. The key target points of injection such as the temporal fossa, piriform recess and masseter region requires a sound understanding of the anatomical landmarks (Fig. 3.2) associated with each area.

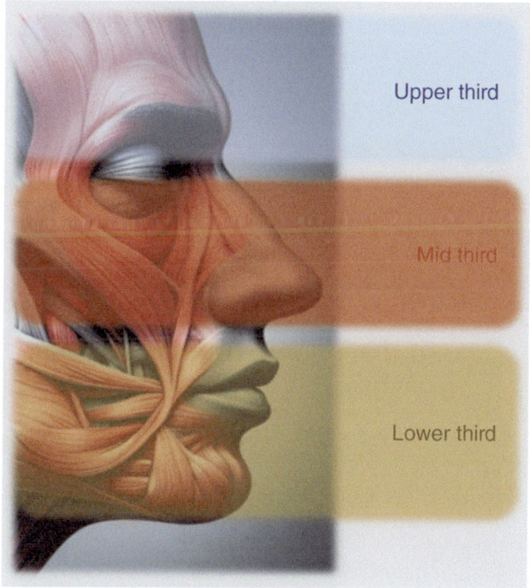

Fig. 3.1 Topographical regions of the face for facial aesthetics refers to the three main anatomical sites of interest during sonographic imaging of the face

K. Malherbe, S. Roberts, *Ultrasound Protocol for Facial Aesthetics*,
https://doi.org/10.1007/978-3-031-75949-9_3

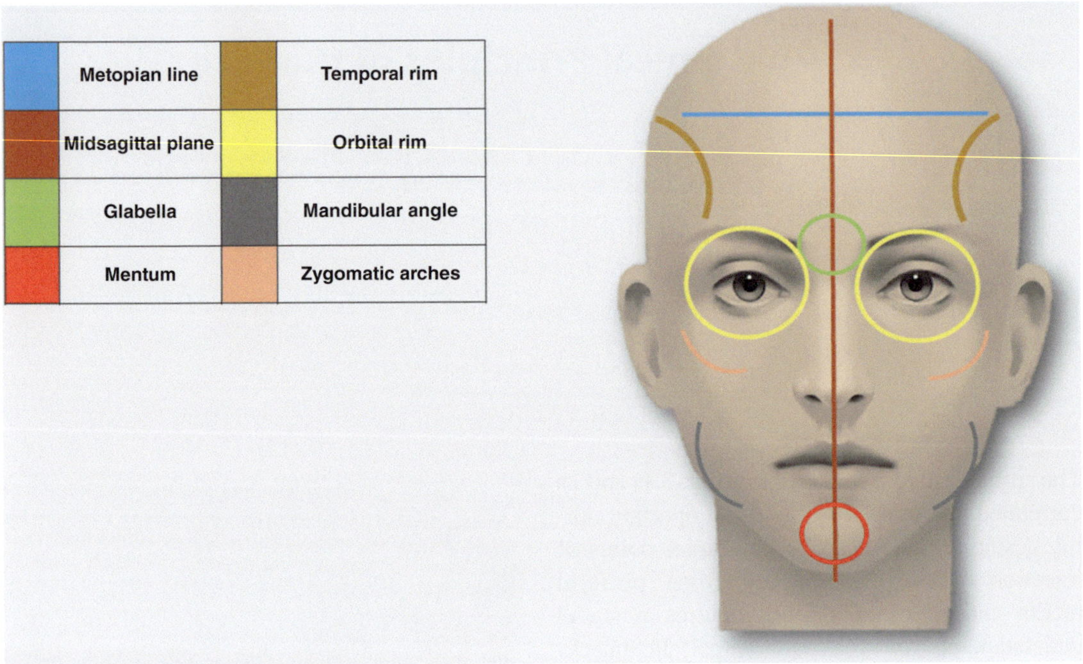

Fig. 3.2 Surface anatomy landmarks

3.1 Injectable Anatomy of the Lower Third of the Face

Muscle	Description	Key information
Masseter muscle	Masseter muscle Is a paired rectangular muscle and consists of both a superficial and deep part. It is one of the masticatory muscles for elevation and protrusion of the mandible as well as support to the temporomandibular joint [1–12].	Origin: Superficial part: maxillary process of zygomatic bone, Inferior border of zygomatic arch (anterior 2/3) Deep part: deep/inferior surface of zygomatic arch (posterior 1/3)
		Insertion: Lateral surface of ramus and angle of mandible
		Action: Elevates and protrudes mandible
		Innervation: Masseteric nerve of mandibular nerve (CN V3) Blood supply: Masseteric artery

Muscle	Description	Key information
Parotid gland	It is the largest of three paired salivary glands, the others being the submandibular and sublingual glands. The parotid main excretory duct (Stenson's duct) projects from the anterior portion of the superficial lobe and runs over the masseter muscle until it reaches its anterior border, from where it turns medially to penetrate the buccinator muscle. It opens into the buccal cavity at the level of the buccal mucosa of the maxillary second molar. The facial nerve courses through the parotid gland, providing motor supply to the muscles of facial expression but does not provide innervation to the gland [2, 5, 7, 8, 11].	Anatomy: It is in the retromandibular fossa, space mainly occupied by this gland. It is bordered superiorly by the zygomatic arch, anteriorly by the masseter muscle, and posteriorly by the sternocleidomastoid muscle. However, the superficial lobe extends anteriorly, covering the mandibular ramus and the posterior area of the masseter muscle. The parotid gland is closely related to two muscles: sternocleidomastoid and masseter. The accessory nerve provides innervation to the sternocleidomastoid muscle [13], which forms the posterior border of the retromandibular fossa
		The parotid glands can be palpated anterior and inferior to the lower half of the ear on the lateral surface of the cheek. They extend inferiorly to the lower border of the mandible and superiorly to the zygomatic arch. Each parotid gland comprises a superficial lobe and a deep lobe divided by the facial nerve and the posterior facial vein. Between the lobes of the gland, there is also fatty tissue that facilitates mandibular movements. The superficial lobe lies lateral to the facial nerve and overlies the lateral surface of the masseter muscle. The deep lobe lies medial to the facial nerve and is situated between the mastoid process of the temporal bone and the mandibular ramus. A fascial capsule called the parotid sheath surrounds the parotid gland
		Action: The parotid gland and the other salivary glands play an essential function in the oral cavity because they secrete saliva, facilitating chewing, swallowing, speaking, and digesting
		Innervation: Sympathetic and parasympathetic fibers innervate the parotid gland. Sympathetic innervation causes vasoconstriction, and parasympathetic innervation, from the glossopharyngeal nerve (CN IX), produces the secretion of saliva [14]. The parasympathetic fibers originate in the inferior salivatory nucleus in the medulla and travel through the jugular foramen to the inferior ganglion. A small branch of the glossopharyngeal nerve, called the tympanic or Jacobsen's nerve, forms the tympanic plexus within the middle ear. These preganglionic fibers become the lesser petrosal nerve and course through the middle cranial fossa before exiting through the foramen ovale. They synapse in the otic ganglion, and the postganglionic parasympathetic fibers join the auriculotemporal nerve to innervate the parotid gland to secrete saliva. Blood supply: The external carotid artery provides blood supply to the parotid. It bifurcates into two terminal branches, the superficial temporal artery, and the maxillary artery. The superficial temporal artery gives off the transverse facial artery, which runs anteriorly between the zygoma and parotid duct and supplies the parotid duct, parotid gland, and masseter muscle. The maxillary artery supplies the infratemporal fossa and the pterygopalatine fossa after exiting the medial portion of the parotid [14]. Finally, the retromandibular vein - which forms from the confluence of the superficial temporal and maxillary veins - provides venous outflow for the parotid.

Muscle	Description	Key information
Risorius muscle	Risorius muscle has a very variable form, ranging from a fleshy slender fascicle to a broad thin superficial fan. Risorius is found in the superficial layer of the facial muscles, coursing over the projection of the line between the alveolar processes of the maxilla and mandible. It is contained in the superficial fascia of the cheek, overlying the masseter muscle and the buccopharyngeal fascia that separates it from the buccinator muscle. Passing between the risorius and buccinator muscle is the facial artery giving off one of its major branches, the superior labial artery. It may seem that the risorius is a continuation of the platysma, but risorius only sometimes receives the upper muscle fibers of the platysma. The proximal region of risorius is related to the parotid gland and parotid duct, which pierces the buccinator muscle into the oral cavity. As it approaches the oral commissure, it contributes to the formation of the modiolus by blending with the zygomaticus major superiorly, with the depressor anguli oris inferiorly and the orbicularis oris laterally [1, 3, 5, 10, 15–17].	Origin: It has several origin points which are sometimes inconsistent and include the zygomatic arch, parotid fascia, fascia over the masseter anterior to the parotid gland, fascia enclosing the platysma and fascia over the mastoid process. Insertion: From these origin points, the muscle fibers of risorius converge medially taking an almost horizontal course towards the oral commissure where it converges to help form a dense, mobile, fibromuscular mass called the modiolus. Action: As the risorius contracts in an outward and upward motion, the muscle pulls the angle of the mouth laterally. Thereby, it aids in producing facial expressions, either solely or in conjunction with other facial muscles, such as smiling, smirking, grinning, frowning and others. Innervation: Buccal branch of facial nerve (CN VII) Blood supply: Risorius muscle is mainly supplied by the superior labial artery, given off by the facial artery as it passes deep to the risorius and superficial to the buccinator. Venous blood is drained by the facial vein, also running deep to the risorius; and the transverse facial vein.
Depressor Anguli oris muscle	Depressor anguli oris originates from the oblique line and mental tubercle of the mandible located on the anterior aspect of the bone. The muscle fibers converge into a narrow fascicle running superiorly towards the oral commissure. It then blends with other muscles that insert into the modiolus. Some fibers of the depressor anguli oris muscle can continue below its origin point at the mental tubercle and cross the midline to blend with the contralateral fibers. These particular fibers form the transversus menti muscle, also called the "mental sling" [9].	Origin: From the oblique line and mental tubercle of the mandible. Insertion: Inserts at the modiolus Action: Assists in dropping of the mouth angle and opening mouth during mastication/speech. Innervation: Marginal and buccal branches of the facial nerve CN VII Blood supply: Depressor anguli oris is supplied by the inferior labial and mental arteries, which are branches of the facial artery and maxillary artery, respectively. The venous blood is drained through the facial vein into the internal jugular vein.
Depressor labii inferioris muscle	Is a small quadrilateral shaped muscle. Previously referred to as quadratus labii inferioris muscle. It arises from the oblique line of the mandible between the symphysis and the mental foramen and moves supero medial onto the integument of the lower lip. The fibers blend with orbicularis oris muscle and contralateral fibers of depressor labii inferioris muscle, continuing with platysma fibers [12].	Origin: Oblique line of mandible Insertion: Integument of the lower lip Action: Depression of lower lip facial animation Innervation: Marginal mandibular nerve branch of the facial nerve. Blood supply: Inferior labial branch of facial artery and mental branch of maxillary artery.

Muscle	Description	Key information
Mentalis	The mentalis muscle is a paired central muscle of the lower lip. It is sometimes referred to as the "pouting muscle" due to raising of the lower lip, producing wrinkles [1–12].	Origin: Mental protuberance near the midline of the mandible.
		Insertion: Soft tissue of the skin and chin
		Action: The mentalis muscle causes a weak upward-inward movement of the soft tissue complex of the chin. This raises the central portion of the lower lip. With regards to lip incompetence, the mentalis muscle contraction can bring temporary but strained oral competence. In conjunction with the orbicularis oris muscle, the mentalis muscle allows pouting of the lip. Externally, the mentalis muscle contraction causes wrinkling and dimpling of the skin on the chin, as used in expressions of doubt or displeasure.
		Innervation: Mandibular branch of Facial nerve Blood supply: Facial artery
Orbicularis oris muscle	Orbicularis oris muscle, also known as musculus orbicularis oris is a complex, multi-layered muscle which attaches through a thin, superficial musculoaponeurotic system to the dermis of the lips and serves as an attachment site for other peri-oral facial muscles. This muscle may be regarded as a single muscle anatomically, but functionally it acts independently or together with other facial muscles of expression. It has neither a bony nor tendinous origin [9].	Origin: Medial aspect of maxilla and mandible, perioral skin, muscles and modiolus
		Insertion: Skin and mucous membrane of lips
		Action: Closes mouth, compresses and protrudes lips
		Innervation: Buccal branch of facial nerve Blood supply: Superior and inferior labial artery (branches of facial artery) Mental and infraorbital artery (branches of maxillary artery) Transverse facial artery (branch of the superficial temporal artery)

3.2 Injectable Anatomy of the Midface

Zygomaticus major and minor muscle	Zygomaticus major and minor muscles are a paired muscle complex lying parallel to each in the cheek area. The zygomaticus major muscle is classified as a buccolabial muscle. Upon muscle activation it assists in creating facial animation related to smiling [1–12].	Origin: Major: Lateral surface of zygomatic bone Minor: Lateral surface of zygomatic bone
		Insertion: Major: Modiolus Minor: Skin and lateral muscles of the lip
		Action: Major: Elevates angle of mouth upward and laterally Minor: Pulls upper lip backward, upward, and laterally Deepens and elevates nasolabial sulcus
		Innervation: Major: Zygomatic and Buccal branches of facial nerve (CN VII) Minor: Buccal branch of facial nerve (CN VII) Blood supply: Major: Superior labial artery of facial artery Minor: Superior labial artery of facial artery

Levator labii superioris alaeque nasalis (LLSAN)	The levator labii superioris alaeque nasi (Latin: musculus levator labii superioris alaeque nasi) is a muscle of facial expression that widens the nostril and elevates the upper lip, producing the facial expression associated with snarling, sometimes referred to as the "Elvis Presley" muscle. It is classified as the nasal facial muscle.	Origin: Frontal process of maxilla
		Insertion: Skin of ala of nose and upper lip
		Action: Dilates nostril. Elevates ala of nose and upper lip
		Innervation: Zygomatic branch of facial nerve (CN VII) Blood supply: Facial artery, infraorbital artery of maxillary artery
Nasalis muscle	Nasalis is a paired muscle that covers the dorsum of the nose. It consists of two parts: alar and transverse. The alar part is also called dilator naris posterior, and the transverse part is known also as the compressor naris. Together with procerus muscle, levator labii superioris alaeque nasi and depressor septi muscles, nasalis belongs to the nasal group of facial muscles.	Origin: Transverse part: covers the dorsum of the nose. It originates from the maxilla, attaching superolateral to the incisive fossa. Its fibers then course superomedial, expanding into a thin aponeurosis at the bridge of the nose. Via this aponeurosis, the muscle inserts at the dorsum of the nose by blending with its counterpart from the opposite side. Alar part: Comprises the nostrils. It originates from the frontal process of maxilla, just superior to the lateral incisor. After a short super anterior course, it inserts to the skin of ala, superior to the lateral crus of major alar cartilage. Here, some fibers blend with the transverse part of nasalis
		Insertion: Transverse part: via the aponeurosis, it inserts at the dorsum of the nose by blending with its counterpart from the opposite side. Alar part: Inserts to the skin of ala, superior to the lateral crus of major alar cartilage. Here, some fibers blend with the transverse part of the nasalis.
		Action: The transverse part of nasalis compresses the nasal aperture, hence its other name compressor naris. The alar part dilates the nostrils as it pulls the ala laterally, thus its name dilator naris posterior. All these actions of nasalis normally happen prior to each inspiration, to prevent the external nasal valve from collapsing. This function of nasalis is even more notable during deep breathing when these movements are more obvious, as well as in affective emotional states such as anger.
		Innervation Branches of the facial nerve Blood supply Facial artery and infraorbital branch of the maxillary artery.
Orbicularis oculi muscle	The orbicularis oculi is a circular-shaped facial muscle located around the opening of the eye. This muscle is classified as the circumorbital and palpebral muscle. Among other functions, the orbicularis oculi muscle is involved in closing the eyelid. The orbicularis oculi are composed of three parts - orbital, palpebral and lacrimal. The orbital part lies circularly around the orbital opening. The palpebral part is situated in the upper and lower eyelids, while the lacrimal part lies most deeply [1–12].	Origin It arises from the nasal part of the frontal bone, from the frontal process of the maxilla, anterior to the lacrimal groove, and from the anterior surface and borders of a short fibrous band, the medial palpebral ligament. From this origin, the fibers are directed laterally, forming a broad and thin layer, which occupies the eyelids or palpebrae, surrounding the circumference of the orbit, and spreads over the temple, and downward on the cheek.
		Insertion This muscle inserts onto the lateral palpebral raphe and superior and inferior tarsal plates, which are also connected to the orbital rim and contribute to the overall structure and function of the eyelids.
		Action: The orbicularis oculi muscle closes the eyelids and assists in pumping the tears from the eye into the nasolacrimal duct system. The orbital section of the orbicularis oculi is more involved in the voluntary closure of the eyelid, such as with winking and forced squeezing. Palpebral part – gently closes the eyelids. Lacrimal part – involved in the drainage of tears. Orbital part – tightly closes the eyelids.
		Innervation: Temporal and zygomatic branches of the facial nerve Blood supply: Branches of superficial temporal, maxillary, facial and ophthalmic arteries.

Temporal muscle	The temporoparietal fascia (TPF) lies under the skin and subcutaneous tissue over the temporal fossa. It is also known as the superficial temporal fascia. It is continuous with the superficial musculoaponeurotic system (SMAS) that is inferior to the zygomatic arch. These two structures are continuous with the platysma muscle in the neck, creating a unified fascia layer from the scalp to the clavicle. The temporoparietal fascia joins the orbicularis oculi and frontalis muscles anteriorly and the occipitalis muscle posteriorly It is approximately 2–3 mm thick. The layers from the skin to the cranium from superficial to deep in this region are as follows: Skin Subcutaneous tissue Temporoparietal fascia (superficial temporal fascia) Innominate fascia Deep temporal fascia (divides into a deep and superficial layer) Temporalis muscle Pericranium Cranium The deep temporal fascia splits into a deep and superficial layer before it inserts into the superior aspect of the zygomatic arch. The superficial temporal fat pad divides these two layers. A proper understanding of the anatomy surrounding the temporoparietal fascia is essential for surgical considerations as it can serve as donor tissue for reconstruction. Additionally, a thorough knowledge of the temporoparietal fascia's relation to surrounding neurovascular structures is integral to safe surgical dissections in this area.	Origin: The temporalis muscle originates from the temporal plane below the superior temporal line of the parietal bone and the deep surface of the temporal fascia. Insertion: The temporalis forms a tendon that inserts onto the coronoid process of the mandible. Action: Upon activation, the temporalis muscle elevates the mandible. It also can retract the mandible by pulling it backward with its posterior fibers. Innervation: The temporalis is innervated by the deep temporal nerve, a branch of the mandibular division of the trigeminal nerve (CN V3). Blood supply: The temporalis is provided with the arterial blood by the deep temporal branches of the maxillary artery and middle temporal branches of the superficial temporal artery.
Retaining ligaments of the midface	The orbicularis retaining ligaments are responsible for forming the superior and inferior boundaries of the orbital compartments of the upper and lower lid, as well as the prezygomatic space. They also overlap with the boundaries of the superficial fat compartments of the face, such as the nasolabial and medial fat compartments, which together form the malar fat pad. This structure is important in midfacial aging and can be elevated and repositioned for aesthetic enhancement. The zygomatic ligaments overlap with the superficial superior cheek septum, separating the lateral orbital compartment from the middle fat compartment. The masseteric cutaneous ligaments also overlap with the septum, separating the middle and medial fat compartments. The platysma-auricular ligament corresponds to the plane between the lateral temporal cheek compartment and the postauricular fat compartment. The mandibular ligament forms the anterior border of the inferior jowl fat compartment, while the mandibular septum separates the superior and inferior jowl fat compartments. Facial aging is a process characterized by soft tissue descent and volumetric deflation, with the role of retaining ligaments in this process being unclear. Some authors suggest that laxity of the ligaments results in laxity and descent of the soft tissue they support, while others suggest that the ligaments remain relatively strong while unsupported tissue descends with time, leading to "stigmata" of facial aging, manifested in bulges and grooves. The nasojugal groove and its lateral extension, the palpebromalar groove, are notable signs of aging. As the orbital septum attenuates with age, the periorbital fat bulges anteriorly against the septum and inferiorly against the orbicularis retaining ligament. This bulge, combined with volumetric deflation in the upper cheek, leads to accentuation and visibility of the orbicularis retaining ligament at the lid-cheek junction. The medial limb of the zygomatic cutaneous ligaments contributes to the formation of the mid cheek groove through cutaneous extensions. Bulging and ptosis of this space with age form malar bags and festoons. Another classic stigma of facial aging is the formation of jowls, formed by the descent of the premasseteric space over the lower portion of the masseter. The superior and inferior jowl fat compartments descend, and the mandibular ligament limits its anterior extension. Another unique aspect of the mandibular ligament is its subcutaneous extension, which can cause skin indentation with aging. Failure to recognize and correct this deformity can lead to patient dissatisfaction after facelift surgery [5]	

3.3 Injectable Facial Anatomy of the Upper Face

Frontalis muscle	The frontalis muscle covers the forehead and skull. Recent literature considers frontalis conjoint to occipitofrontalis muscle. The occipitofrontalis is composed of two muscle bellies: frontalis and occipitalis, which are attached and encased by dense connective tissue called the epicranial aponeurosis or galea aponeurotica. The occipital part of the occipitofrontalis muscle moves the scalp forwards, and the frontalis part lifts the brows and moves the anterior scalp backward. When the frontalis muscle contracts, the vertical fibers pull the skin of the eyebrows upward. The superficial musculoaponeurotic system (SMAS) continues above the zygomatic arch and includes the temporoparietal fascia (as it blends into the galea) and the frontalis muscle as part of the SMAS. The antagonist muscles to the frontalis muscle are the orbicularis oculi, corrugator supercilli and procerus muscles. The frontalis muscle has no bony attachments. The corrugator muscle is deep to the frontalis and the orbicularis muscles and has a bony origin from the medial orbital rim. Frontalis muscle action produces horizontal forehead lines. Four types of forehead lines have been described: 1. Full, straight lines that run across the whole forehead (45%) 2. Gull wing-shaped lines with a central depression and lateral elevation (30%) 3. Short central horizontal lines over the middle of the forehead but few or no lines laterally (10%) 4. Lateral straight lines as two columns formed on the lateral aspect of the forehead with no central lines (15%) [1–3, 5, 12]	Origin: It originates posteriorly from the galea aponeurotica, which corresponds with the hairline on the surface. Insertion: Inferomedial, the muscle interdigitates with fibers of procerus muscle, while more inferolateral, it has attachments to the orbicularis oculi and corrugator muscles Action: The frontalis muscle is responsible for raising the eyebrows and wrinkling the skin on the forehead. It helps with facial expressions Innervation: The muscles of facial expression receive nerve supply from cranial nerve VII (the facial nerve), which separates into five main branches: temporal, zygomatic, buccal, marginal mandibular, and cervical. The facial nerve exits the skull at the stylomastoid foramen and its temporal branch crosses over the zygomatic arch, passes through the areolar tissue on the surface of the temporal fascia, and subsequently enters the frontalis muscle to provide its deep innervation. Three branches of the temporal nerve, the anterior, middle, and posterior, are responsible for innervating the orbicularis oculi, frontalis, and the corrugator muscles Blood supply: The frontalis muscle receives its blood supply from branches of both the internal and external carotid arteries. The supratrochlear and supraorbital arteries supply the muscle from the inferior margin after they exit the orbit and travel up the forehead. The supraorbital artery can exit from the supraorbital notch/foramen, while the supratrochlear artery exits more medially from the orbit. They are both branches of the ophthalmic artery, which is a branch of the internal carotid artery. The superficial arteries supply the muscle, galea, and skin, while the deeper layer supplies the periosteum. The supratrochlear and supraorbital arteries supply a bulk of the blood medially, and the frontal branch, which comes off of the superficial temporal artery, supplies the muscle more laterally. The arteries form an anastomosis with one another to form a highly vascularized network

Procerus muscle	The procerus muscle is a pyramidal-shaped muscle of facial expression part of the glabella/nasal complex. The procerus muscle is derived from the second pharyngeal arch, innervated by branches of the facial nerve, and supplied by the facial artery via the external carotid artery. The structure and functionality of the procerus muscle and the associated glabellar complex are of clinical importance in cosmetic and surgical procedures, including botulinum toxin injection, injectable fillers, and blepharoplasty	Origin: The procerus muscle is a pyramidal-shaped muscle arising from the fascia of the superior nasal region, near the junction of the nasal bones, and the superolateral nasal cartilage. [1] The procerus muscle fibers run superiorly and merge with the frontalis muscle
		Insertion: Skin of glabella, fibers of frontal belly of occipitofrontalis muscle
		Action: Depresses medial end of eyebrow, wrinkles skin over the nasion
		Innervation: Temporal, lower zygomatic or buccal branches of facial nerve (CN VII) Blood supply: Angular and lateral nasal branches of facial artery
Corrugator supercilli muscle	Small narrow facial muscle found along the medial edge of the eyebrow. Classified as a circumorbital and palpebral muscle [1–3, 5, 12]	Origin: Medial part of superciliary arch
		Insertion: Skin above middle part of eyebrow
		Action: Pulls skin of eyebrow downward and medially, producing vertical wrinkles of forehead
		Innervation: Temporal branch of facial nerve Blood supply: Branches of superficial temporal and ophthalmic arteries

3.4 Vascular Anatomy of the Face Related to Filler Injection

The facial artery (Fig. 3.3) supplies blood to the superficial facial anatomy structures. It is a branch of the external carotid artery. The omohyoid muscle's superior belly, the sternocleidomastoid muscle, and the digastric muscle's posterior belly create the carotid triangle, which gives origin to the facial artery. The facial artery starts deep within the platysma and ends abruptly at the surface. This artery can extend further during face motions like mastication because of its winding path. Traveling deep to the posterior belly of the digastric and stylohyoid muscles, the vessel passes over the face.

It then proceeds along the submandibular gland's posterior surface. The artery runs along the masseter's anterior inferior border before curving upward across the mandible's body. You may feel the pulse of the facial artery as it passes through your jaw. The angular artery, which ends at the medial canthus of the eye, ascends the side of the nose, and continues superiorly at an oblique angle across the cheek towards the oral commissure.

Numerous branches of the facial artery nourish various structures. The muscles located deep to this vasculature are the buccinator and levator anguli oris, which are supplied by the facial artery. The artery might go over the levator labii superioris in the usual version or through it. The levator veli palatini, masseter, mentalis, mylohyoid, nasalis, palatoglossus, palatopharyngeal, platysma, procerus, risorius, styloglossus, and the transverse section of the nasalis are among the other muscles fed by the facial artery. Additionally, it nourishes the submandibular gland, pterygoid muscles, digastric muscles, soft palate, and palatine tonsils [14, 18–21].

Before continuing into the face, the cervical branch of the facial artery gives rise to four additional arteries. The tonsillar branch, glandular

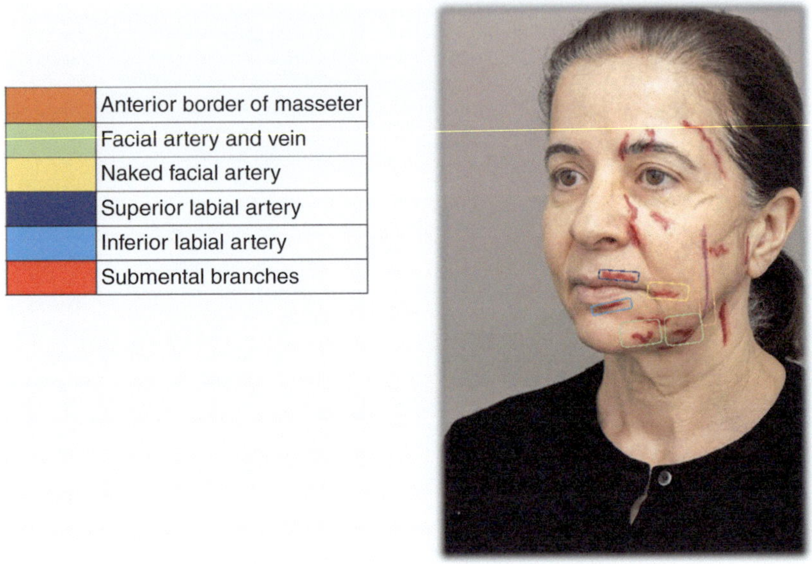

Fig. 3.3 Facial artery course using a systematic point system
From the anterior border of the masseter the facial artery course follows systematically with the musculature in this region

branches, submental artery, and ascending palatine artery are the vessels of the cervical branches. The lower labial artery, superior labial artery, lateral nasal branch (to the nasalis), and angular artery are the four principal facial vessels that emerge from the facial artery trunk. The facial artery's terminal portion is called the angular artery.

The deep superior cervical lymph nodes are close to the facial artery's origin. As the facial artery runs superficially toward the face, the submandibular lymph nodes are located next to it. The submandibular and face lymph nodes stay deep to this vessel as the artery crests over the mandibular body. Deep into the proximal facial artery runs the hypoglossal nerve. It is also usual for the facial artery to run deep to the facial nerve's marginal mandibular branch.

Facial artery reconstruction is involved in facial operations. For different types of flaps, such as local, regional, or free flaps, it can serve as the vascular supply. The buccinator myomucosal, submental, platysma muscle, nasolabial, and facial artery Musculo mucosal flaps are among the frequently used flaps that include the facial artery. These kinds of reconstructive operations can be carried out after heel and neck tumors have been removed. The face artery has strong pulsatile flow and can deliver enough blood through transplanted tissue.

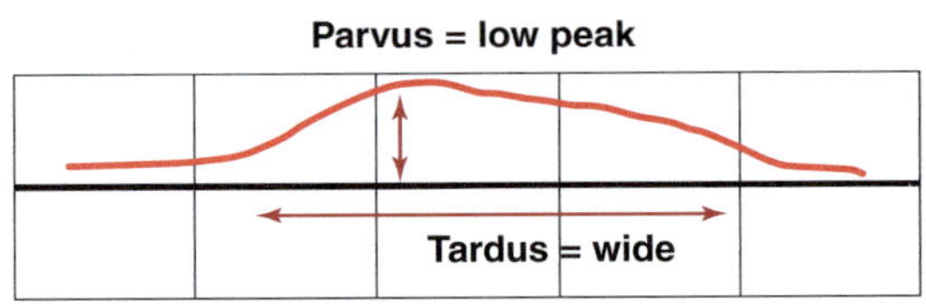

Fig. 3.4 Differences in spectral tracing in pathological examples
Principle of waveform pre, intra and post stenosis measurements

Complications from a variety of surgical operations may have an impact on the facial artery. It is critical to prevent damage to the facial artery. It is therefore best to refrain from unduly retracting in this field. Excision of the submandibular gland may also result in hemorrhage from the facial artery. It may be necessary to ligate the facial artery to repair mandible fractures using external methods. To ensure that future surgeons have a reference for this, thorough documentation should be provided in the operation note if necessary (Fig. 3.4). In case of bleeding from the facial artery, the mandibular angle should be directly compressed until the bleeding source is located and managed.

Recognizing the proximity of certain nerves, such as the hypoglossal nerve, to the face artery is crucial while performing surgical treatments. To reduce post-operative problems,

Fig. 3.5 Spectral tracing values for arteries of the face Resistive Index (RI) and Peak Systolic Velocity (PSV) rates for arteries of the face

Artery	PSV (cm/s)	RI
Facial	45.31	0.81
Submental	21.07	0.79
Inferior labial	27.99	0.77
Superior labial	27.38	0.72
Angular	20.73	0.65
Mental	23.05	0.78
Infraorbital	15.55	0.75
Superficial temporal	42.09	0.79
Transverse facial	21.38	0.74
Total average	**27.17**	**0.75**

these structures must be recognized early and maintained.

The facial artery's superficial route makes it possible to feel it's pulse at the masseter muscle's anterior inferior angle against the mandibular bone [19, 22].

Figure 3.5 demonstrates abnormal spectral tracing seen during arterial occlusion, the first image A refers to a tardus parvus waveform (Fig. 3.5), the image shows stenosis with diminished peak systolic amplitude and prolonged systolic acceleration evident in delayed systolic upstroke and rounded systolic peak. Image B refers to the typical flow pattern before, during and after an arterial occlusion. Image B is important as this allows the clinician to have a better understanding of the origin of the occlusion, so that the use of hyaluronidase is target to the area of direct occlusion and not distal to the affected site.

It is documented that in approximately 70% of cases of internal carotid artery occlusion, there is a significant pulse of the angular artery, which is the terminal branch of the facial artery. Anastomotic channels are present between the dorsal nasal and supratrochlear branches of the ophthalmic artery on the internal carotid side and the angular branch of the facial artery and the medial branches of the infraorbital artery on the external carotid side. The fact that this result is typical in 1 out of 10 persons over 55 who have had chronic hypertension, however, limits its diagnostic value [19].

One risk factor for embolic events that result in ischemia injury is atherosclerosis of the common carotid artery. A facial artery vascular impairment could occur if there is a deficit in the superficial facial musculature. A distal branch of the facial artery may sustain ischemia due to a common carotid embolism. But carotid artery atherosclerosis seldom results in this [14].

The measurement of the PSV And RI rates of arteries of the face provides an additional dimension to the standard measurement values expected and when arterial occlusion is suspected. Figure 3.5 is the only known study, with a limited sample population of 40 patients which provided a standard mean for each of the arteries to be used. In carotid artery assessment, a standard measurement is commonly used to determine the presence of intra-arterial pathology [14, 19, 23, 24].

References

1. Wu WT, Chang KV, Chang HC, Chen LR, Kuan CH, Kao JT, et al. Ultrasound imaging of the facial muscles and relevance with Botulinum toxin injections: a pictorial essay and narrative review. Toxins (Basel). 2022;14(2) https://doi.org/10.3390/toxins14020101.
2. Arlette JP, Trotter MJ. Anatomic location of hyaluronic acid filler material injected into nasolabial fold: a histologic study. Dermatologic Surg. 2008;34(Suppl 1):S56–62. https://doi.org/10.1111/j.1524-4725.2008.34244.x. discussion S-3
3. Lee HJ, Jung SJ, Kim ST, Kim HJ. Ultrasonographic considerations for safe and efficient Botulinum neurotoxin injection in Masseteric hypertrophy. Toxins (Basel). 2021;13(1) https://doi.org/10.3390/toxins13010028.
4. Singh V. Textbook of anatomy head, neck, and brain. 2nd ed. Elsevier; 2014.

5. Haddock NT, Saadeh PB, Boutros S, Thorne CH. The tear trough and lid/cheek junction: anatomy and implications for surgical correction. Plast Reconstr Surg. 2009;123(4):1332–40. https://doi.org/10.1097/PRS.0b013e31819f2b36.
6. Van de Graaf KM. Human anatomy. McGraw Hill Higher Education; 2001.
7. Drake RL, Vogl W, Mitchell AWM, Gray H. Gray's anatomy for students. 3rd ed. Philadephia: Churchill Livingstone/Elsevier; 2015.
8. Tamura B. Facial anatomy view for aesthetic botulinum toxin injection. In: Daily routine in cosmetic dermatology; 2019. p. 1–8.
9. Moore M, Dalley KL, Arthur F. Clinically oriented anatomy. 2nd ed. Wolwers Kluter; 2017.
10. Jain P, Raphee M. Anatomy of the orbicularis oris muscle. Treasure Island Publishers; 2023.
11. Chason H.M. Anatomy of the head and neck. Treasure Island Publishers. 2022;
12. Watanabe K, Shoja MM, Loukas M, Tubbs RS. Anatomy for plastic surgery of the face, head, and neck. 1st ed. Thieme Publishers; 2016.
13. Gerr A [Internet]. Anisotropy as most important pitfall in ultrasound imaging. 2023. Available from: www.sonoskills.com.
14. Kim SH. Interpretation of peripheral arterial and venous Doppler waveforms: a consensus statement from the Society for Vascular Medicine and Society for vascular ultrasound. Vasc Med. 2020;25(5):484–506.
15. Bhoi S, Chandra A, Galwankar S. Ultrasound-guided nerve blocks in the emergency department. J Emerg Trauma Shock. 2010;3(1):82–8. https://doi.org/10.4103/0974-2700.58655.
16. Sundaram H, Signorini M, Liew S, Trindade de Almeida AR, Wu Y, Vieira Braz A, et al. Global Aesthetics Consensus: Botulinum Toxin Type A--Evidence-Based Review, Emerging Concepts, and Consensus Recommendations for Aesthetic Use, Including Updates on Complications. Plast Reconstr Surg 2016; 137(3):518e-529e. https://doi.org/10.1097/01.prs.0000475758.63709.23.
17. Buchanan PJ, Grossman JAI, Price AE, Reddy C, Chopan M, Chim H. The use of botulinum toxin injection for brachial plexus birth injuries: a systematic review of the literature. Hand (NY). 2019;14(2):150–4. https://doi.org/10.1177/1558944718760038.
18. Rayess HM, Svider PF, Hanba C, Patel VS, DeJoseph LM, Carron M, et al. A cross-sectional analysis of adverse events and litigation for injectable fillers. JAMA Facial Plast Surg. 2018;20(3):207–14. https://doi.org/10.1001/jamafacial.2017.1888.
19. Tucunduva MJ, Tucunduva-Neto R, Saieg M, Costa AL, de Freitas C. Vascular mapping of the face: B-mode and doppler ultrasonography study. Med Oral Patol Oral Cir Bucal. 2016;21(2):e135–41. https://doi.org/10.4317/medoral.20754.
20. Beleznay K, Humphries S, Carruthers JDA, Carruthers A. Vascular compromise from soft tissue augmentation: experience with 12 cases and recommendations for optimal outcomes. J Clin Aesthet Dermatol. 2014;7(9):37–43.
21. Sito G, Manzoni V, Sommariva R. Vascular complications after facial filler injection: a literature review and meta-analysis. J Clin Aesth Dermatol. 2019;12(6):E65–72.
22. Alam M, Dover JS. Management of complications and sequelae with temporary injectable fillers. Plast Reconstr Surg. 2007;120(6 Suppl):98S–105S. https://doi.org/10.1097/01.prs.0000248859.14788.60.
23. Shah A, Irshad A. Sonography doppler flow imaging instrumentation. Statpearls; 2024.
24. Key R [Internet]. Doppler Flow Imaging and Spectral Analysis 2017 [5 September 2022]. Available from: https://www.radiologykey.com/spectralanalysis.

4 Clinical Indications for Facial Aesthetic Ultrasound

The use of ultrasound is gaining more interest among aesthetic physicians worldwide. Ultrasound allows aesthetic physicians and radiologists real-time assessment of the patient during the initial consultation, immediate pre-treatment, assisting with treatment, and assessing the patient post-treatment [35].

4.1 Pre-Treatment Indications

- Assessment of the vasculature of the upper, mid, and lower face before filler treatment, in high-risk zones
- Determine the origin and route of vascular flow in the target treatment area for both the internal and external carotid artery origins.

NB: It's important to note that the arteries of the face are complex, tortuous, and small in diameter (clinical correlation is advised before treatment).

- Assess the depth of the injection during a dynamic ultrasound assessment.
- For determining the depth of injection, for regions of high vascular compromise risk, such as the temple, forehead, and nose.
- Assessment of the presence of aging filler treatments.
  - Various types of filler can be discerned using B-mode ultrasound and shear wave elastography imaging.
  - Filler aging relates to the echogenicity of the filler bolus site from anechoic to a more heterogeneous appearance.
- Clinical appearance of asymmetry of the face; to assess anatomical variance that is present using ultrasound.
  - For patients presenting with, for example, an asymmetrical masseter region, dynamic sonographic assessment of the various muscle bellies of the masseter muscle will assist in determining key target areas for treatment [1–41].

4.2 Post-Treatment Indications

- Vascular complication following filler treatment for referral for US-guided injection of hyaluronidase.
  - Assessment to determine flow impedance using spectral Doppler imaging.
  - Determine the presence of filler around vascular compromise.
  - Assessment of post-hyaluronidase treatment to confirm vascular flow has improved.
- To assess the correct depth and placement of fillers in key target areas such as the temple, tear trough and piriform recess.
- During a follow-up assessment of botulinum toxin in areas of asymmetry, such as the masseter muscles, the dynamic sonographic con-

K. Malherbe, S. Roberts, *Ultrasound Protocol for Facial Aesthetics*,
https://doi.org/10.1007/978-3-031-75949-9_4

traction would assist in determining effective treatment post-injection with clinical correlation [1–4, 6–8, 10–19, 21–27, 30, 32–36, 38–41].

4.3 Limitations of Use for Facial Aesthetics

- The differentiation of various types of filler products using ultrasound is limiting. Alternate modalities like magnetic resonance imaging are advised [1].

References

1. Wu WT, Chang KV, Chang HC, Chen LR, Kuan CH, Kao JT, et al. Ultrasound imaging of the facial muscles and relevance with Botulinum toxin injections: a pictorial essay and narrative review. Toxins (Basel). 2022;14(2) https://doi.org/10.3390/toxins14020101.
2. Zetlaoui PJ, Gauthier E, Benhamou D. Ultrasound-guided scalp nerve blocks for neurosurgery: a narrative review. Anaesth Crit Care Pain Med. 2020;39(6):876–82. https://doi.org/10.1016/j.accpm.2020.06.019.
3. Bhoi S, Chandra A, Galwankar S. Ultrasound-guided nerve blocks in the emergency department. J Emerg Trauma Shock. 2010;3(1):82–8. https://doi.org/10.4103/0974-2700.58655.
4. Ryu JH, Shim JH, Yeom JH, Shin WJ, Cho SY, Jeon WJ. Ultrasound-guided greater occipital nerve block with botulinum toxin for patients with chronic headache in the occipital area: a randomized controlled trial. Korean J Anesthesiol. 2019;72(5):479–85. https://doi.org/10.4097/kja.19145.
5. Kim SH. Interpretation of peripheral arterial and venous Doppler waveforms: a consensus statement from the Society for Vascular Medicine and Society for vascular ultrasound. Vasc Med. 2020;25(5):484–506.
6. Gerr A [Internet]. Anisotropy as most important pitfall in ultrasound imaging. 2023. Available from: www.sonoskills.com.
7. Food and Drug Administration. XEOMIN (incobotulinumtoxinA). Silver Spring, MD: FDA; 2010. p. 10.
8. Food and Drug Administration. BOTOX (onabotulinumtoxinA). In: Drug FM, editor. FDA; 1989.
9. Greco GA. Plastic surgery statistics report. Arlington Heights, IL: American Soceity of Plastic Surgeons; 2022.
10. The Aesthetic Soceity. The aesthetic society statistics. Aesthetic Plastic Surgery National Databank, 2021.
11. Sundaram H, Signorini M, Liew S, Trindade de Almeida AR, Wu Y, Vieira Braz A, et al. Global Aesthetics Consensus: Botulinum Toxin Type A--Evidence-Based Review, Emerging Concepts, and Consensus Recommendations for Aesthetic Use, Including Updates on Complications. Plast Reconstr Surg 2016; 137(3):518e-529e. https://doi.org/10.1097/01.prs.0000475758.63709.23.
12. Pikoos TD, Buzwell S, Sharp G, Rossell SL. The zoom effect: exploring the impact of video calling on appearance dissatisfaction and interest in aesthetic treatment during the COVID-19 pandemic. Aesthet Surg J. 2021;41(12):NP2066–75. https://doi.org/10.1093/asj/sjab257.
13. Samizadeh S, De Boulle K. Complications of toxins and fillers in facial aesthetics. Prim Dent J. 2023;12(3):65–72.
14. Malherbe K. Image-guided injection techniques. Pretoria: Boutique Book Publishers; 2023.
15. Beer K. Dermal fillers and combinations of fillers for facial rejuvenation. Dermatol Clin. 2009;27(4):427–32. https://doi.org/10.1016/j.det.2009.08.011.
16. Rayess HM, Svider PF, Hanba C, Patel VS, DeJoseph LM, Carron M, et al. A cross-sectional analysis of adverse events and litigation for injectable fillers. JAMA Facial Plast Surg. 2018;20(3):207–14. https://doi.org/10.1001/jamafacial.2017.1888.
17. Daines SM, Williams EF. Complications associated with injectable soft-tissue fillers: a 5-year retrospective review. JAMA Facial Plast Surg. 2013;15(3):226–31. https://doi.org/10.1001/jamafacial.2013.798.
18. Arlette JP, Trotter MJ. Anatomic location of hyaluronic acid filler material injected into nasolabial fold: a histologic study. Dermatologic Surg. 2008;34(Suppl 1):S56–62. https://doi.org/10.1111/j.1524-4725.2008.34244.x. discussion S-3
19. Tucunduva MJ, Tucunduva-Neto R, Saieg M, Costa AL, de Freitas C. Vascular mapping of the face: B-mode and doppler ultrasonography study. Med Oral Patol Oral Cir Bucal. 2016;21(2):e135–41. https://doi.org/10.4317/medoral.20754.
20. Shah A, Irshad A. Sonography doppler flow imaging instrumentation. Statpearls; 2024.
21. Key R [Internet]. Doppler Flow Imaging and Spectral Analysis 2017 [5 September 2022]. Available from: https://www.radiologykey.com/spectralanalysis.
22. Ambroziak M, Noszczyk B, Pietruski P, Guz W, Paluch L. Elastography reference values of facial skin elasticity. Postepy Dermatol Alergol. 2019;36(5):626–34. https://doi.org/10.5114/ada.2018.77502.
23. Papageorgiou K, Chang HS, Isaacs D, Fiaschetti D, Ang M, Goldberg R. Refining the goals of oculofacial rejuvenation with dynamic ultrasonography. Aesthet Surg J. 2012;32(2):207–19. https://doi.org/10.1177/1090820X11434523.
24. Alam M, Dover JS. Management of complications and sequelae with temporary injectable fillers. Plast Reconstr Surg. 2007;120(6 Suppl):98S–105S. https://doi.org/10.1097/01.prs.0000248859.14788.60.

25. Lee HJ, Jung SJ, Kim ST, Kim HJ. Ultrasonographic considerations for safe and efficient Botulinum neurotoxin injection in Masseteric hypertrophy. Toxins (Basel). 2021;13(1) https://doi.org/10.3390/toxins13010028.
26. Singh V. Textbook of anatomy head, neck, and brain. 2nd ed. Elsevier; 2014.
27. Haddock NT, Saadeh PB, Boutros S, Thorne CH. The tear trough and lid/cheek junction: anatomy and implications for surgical correction. Plast Reconstr Surg. 2009;123(4):1332–40. https://doi.org/10.1097/PRS.0b013e31819f2b36.
28. Van de Graaf KM. Human anatomy. McGraw Hill Higher Education; 2001.
29. Drake RL, Vogl W, Mitchell AWM, Gray H. Gray's anatomy for students. 3rd ed. Philadephia: Churchill Livingstone/Elsevier; 2015.
30. Tamura B. Facial anatomy view for aesthetic botulinum toxin injection. In: Daily routine in cosmetic dermatology; 2019. p. 1–8.
31. Moore M, Dalley KL, Arthur F. Clinically oriented anatomy. 2nd ed. Wolwers Kluter; 2017.
32. Jain P, Raphee M. Anatomy of the orbicularis oris muscle. Treasure Island Publishers; 2023.
33. Chason H.M. Anatomy of the head and neck. Treasure Island Publishers. 2022;
34. Watanabe K, Shoja MM, Loukas M, Tubbs RS. Anatomy for plastic surgery of the face, head, and neck. 1st ed. Thieme Publishers; 2016.
35. Buchanan PJ, Grossman JAI, Price AE, Reddy C, Chopan M, Chim H. The use of botulinum toxin injection for brachial plexus birth injuries: a systematic review of the literature. Hand (NY). 2019;14(2):150–4. https://doi.org/10.1177/1558944718760038.
36. Beleznay K, Humphries S, Carruthers JDA, Carruthers A. Vascular compromise from soft tissue augmentation: experience with 12 cases and recommendations for optimal outcomes. J Clin Aesthet Dermatol. 2014;7(9):37–43.
37. Sito G, Manzoni V, Sommariva R. Vascular complications after facial filler injection: a literature review and meta-analysis. J Clin Aesth Dermatol. 2019;12(6):E65–72.
38. Janis JE, Barker JC, Palettas M. Targeted peripheral nerve-directed onabotulinumtoxin a injection for effective long-term therapy for migraine headache. Plast Reconstr Surg Glob Open. 2017;5(3):e1270. https://doi.org/10.1097/GOX.0000000000001270.
39. Hood K, Ganesh Kumar N, Kaoutzanis C, Higdon KK. Hematomas in aesthetic surgery. Aesthet Surg J. 2018;38(9):1013–25. https://doi.org/10.1093/asj/sjx236.
40. Chandra M, Dara S, Varma R. A case report on botox for neurogenic thoracic outlet syndrome—an alternative to surgery. Ind J Pain. 2022;36(3) https://doi.org/10.4103/ijpn.ijpn_88_21.
41. Turk Boru U, Duman A, Boluk C, Coskun Duman S, Tasdemir M. Botulinum toxin in the treatment of trigeminal neuralgia: 6-month follow-up. Medicine (Baltimore). 2017;96(39):e8133. https://doi.org/10.1097/MD.0000000000008133.

5 Clinical Complications/Pathological Indications Related to Facial Aesthetics

5.1 Vascular Anatomy and Its Implications in Facial Aesthetic Procedures

Understanding the vascular anatomy is paramount in facial aesthetic procedures to ensure safe and successful outcomes. The face is a highly vascularized region, and knowledge of arteries, veins, and their branches is crucial for avoiding complications. This knowledge aids practitioners in selecting appropriate injection sites, avoiding vital vessels, and minimizing the risk of vascular compromise, which can lead to severe complications such as necrosis and blindness [1].

In facial aesthetic procedures, inadvertent injury to facial arteries and veins can result in serious consequences. Injecting dermal fillers or performing surgical procedures in proximity to critical vessels may lead to complications like vascular occlusion, embolism, or hematoma formation. Vascular compromise (Fig. 5.1) can compromise blood flow, causing tissue necrosis, scarring, and even permanent damage. The danger is heightened in areas with anastomoses, where occluding one vessel may redirect blood flow to another, compounding the risk.

Case studies have reported instances of vision loss following facial filler injections, particularly in areas around the eyes and forehead [1–4]. The inadvertent injection into arteries, such as the ophthalmic artery, can cause retinal artery occlusion and result in permanent blindness. Compromising blood supply to facial tissues, often due to filler injections or certain surgical procedures, can lead to ischemia and tissue necrosis. Cases of nasal tip necrosis after rhinoplasty or dermal filler injections have been documented [1, 5–11].

Complications such as vascular embolism have been reported, where filler material inadvertently enters blood vessels and travels to distant parts of the body. This can lead to serious systemic complications, including cardiovascular issues.

Surgical procedures, especially those involving deeper tissues, can pose a risk of damaging facial veins, resulting in hematoma formation. This can lead to localized swelling, pain, and potential complications if not managed appropriately [1, 5–11].

5.1.1 Vascular Compromise in Facial Aesthetics: Signs and Symptoms

Vascular compromise during facial aesthetic treatments can manifest through various signs and symptoms, signaling potential complications. Immediate signs include blanching or pallor of the

Supplementary Information The online version contains supplementary material available at https://doi.org/10.1007/978-3-031-75949-9_5.

K. Malherbe, S. Roberts, *Ultrasound Protocol for Facial Aesthetics*,
https://doi.org/10.1007/978-3-031-75949-9_5

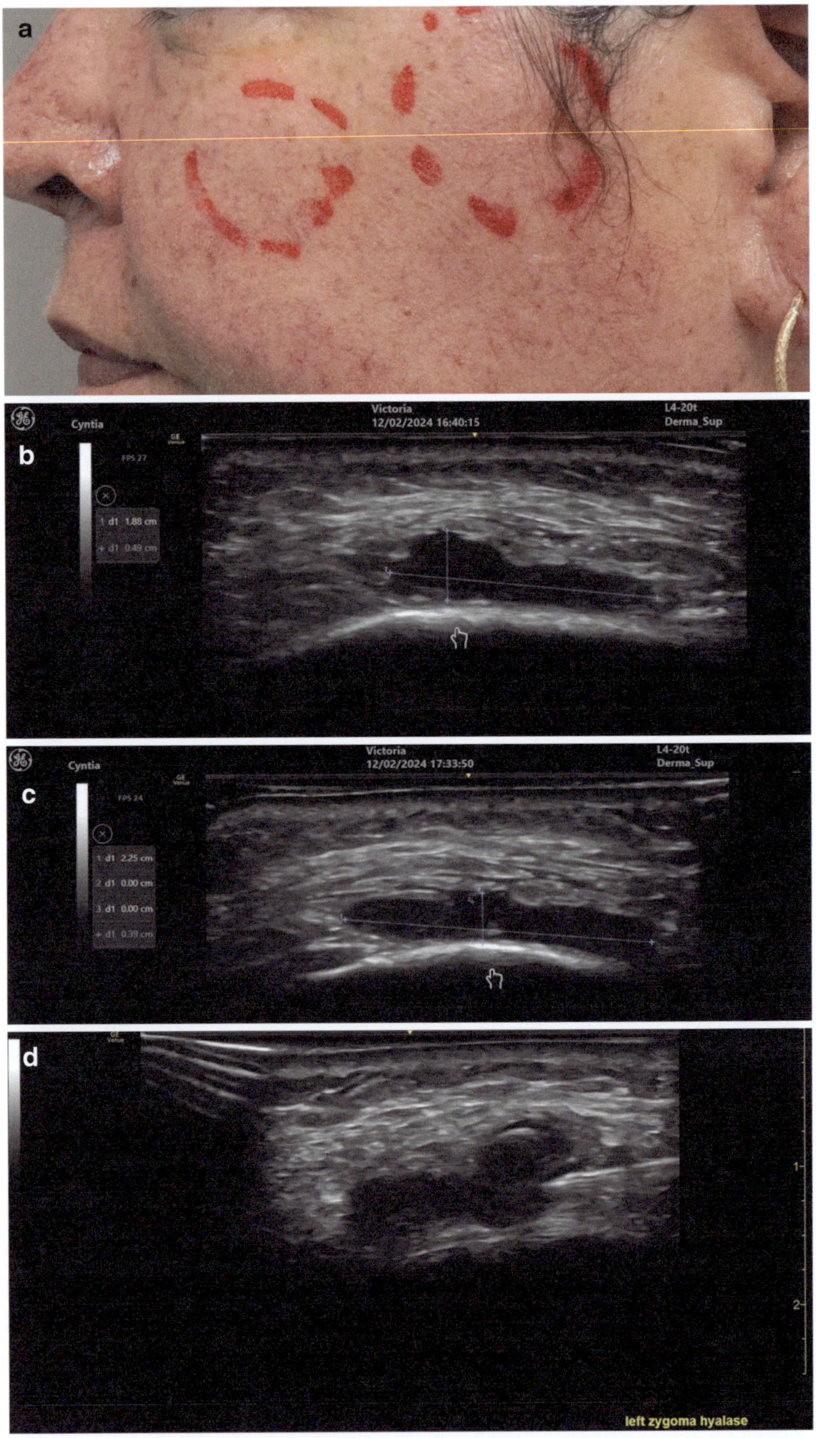

Fig. 5.1 Clinical and ultrasound images of vascular occlusion (Case study 1)
Presentation of a delayed onset nodule in 50-year-old patient, 13 days post hyaluronidase (low density) filler treatment
(**a**) Two separate nodules were present, the first in the prezygomatic space and the 2nd 2 cm posterior
Nodules presented with localized pain and swelling. Initial treatment included antibiotic treatment and oral corticosteroids
(**b**) Ultrasound shows an oval shaped mixed echogenic fluid collection with an echogenic rim/capsule. Surrounding soft tissue appears erythematous, like sonographic appearance of cellulitis formation (cobblestone appearance)
(**c**) Refers to pre-clinical assessment
Serial imaging over 6 week period is suggested to confirm resolvement of nodule
(**d**) refers to live ultrasound video during guided injection of the second smaller nodule, a hyperechoic fluid bolus is noted entering the nodule capsule

skin, mottling, and a dusky appearance. Patients may also experience pain, which can be disproportionate to the procedure, and a feeling of tightness in the treated area. In severe cases, cyanosis and coolness of the skin may occur. Additionally, the absence of expected blanching or bluish hue upon release of pressure during injection points towards vascular compromise [1, 2, 10, 12, 13].

The initial signs of vascular compromise are often noticeable during or immediately after the procedure. Immediate manifestations include sudden pain, skin color changes, and poor capillary refill upon compression. These symptoms require immediate attention to prevent further complications.

Vascular compromise can also lead to delayed complications. Necrosis, or tissue death, may become apparent hours or even days after the procedure. Patients may experience persistent pain, skin ulceration, and scarring. Recognizing delayed manifestations is crucial for timely intervention and management [1, 5–11].

5.1.2 Diagnostic Criteria for Recognizing Vascular Compromise in Clinical Practice

- Careful examination of the treated area is essential. Look for changes in skin color, temperature, and texture.
- Assess capillary refill time and note any asymmetry or abnormal swelling. If the patient reports severe and persistent pain that is disproportionate to the procedure, it may indicate vascular compromise.
- In certain cases, imaging techniques such as ultrasound or Doppler can be employed to assess blood flow and identify any vascular abnormalities.
  - These methods can aid in confirming the diagnosis and assessing the extent of the compromise.
- Consulting with vascular surgeons or other specialists may be necessary for a comprehensive evaluation, especially in complex cases.
  - They can provide expertise in interpreting imaging results and guide appropriate interventions.
- Understanding the patient's medical history, including any pre-existing vascular conditions or previous complications during aesthetic procedures, is crucial (Fig. 5.2).
  - Patients with a history of vascular compromise may be more susceptible, and precautions should be taken.
- Recognizing the signs of vascular compromise is only the first step; a prompt and effective response is critical. Immediate cessation of the procedure, application of warm compresses, and administration of hyaluronidase (if applicable) can be essential in mitigating complications [1, 2, 10, 12, 13].

In conclusion, vigilance and a comprehensive understanding of the signs, immediate and delayed manifestations, and diagnostic criteria for vascular compromise are crucial in the context of facial aesthetic treatments. Early recognition and intervention significantly contribute to minimizing the potential risks and optimizing patient outcomes.

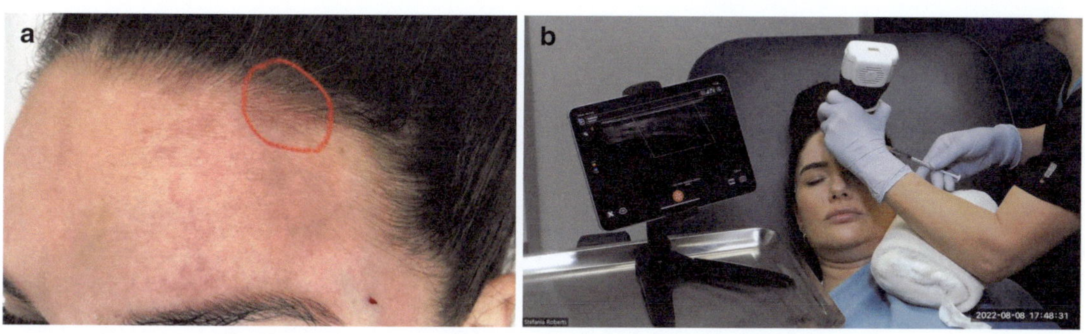

Fig. 5.2 Clinical and ultrasound images of vascular occlusion of superficial temporal artery (Case study 2)
(**a**) 43-year-old female patient presented with signs of vascular occlusion within 24 hours of filler treatment
Note the course of ecchymosis is relevant to Superficial temporal artery course
Following treatment with hyaluronidase 10 500 IU divided into three separate treatment sessions, patient had persistent tingling and burning sensation
(**b**) Live video demonstrates use of ultrasound guidance during hyaluronidase injection. Note the use of sterile technique

5.1.3 Management of Vascular Complications in Facial Aesthetics

A Step-by-Step Guide to Managing Vascular Compromise in Facial Aesthetic Treatments would include factors such as: [5, 7, 8, 11]

Immediate Recognition:	Recognize the signs of vascular compromise during or immediately after the procedure, including changes in skin color, pain, and poor capillary refill.
Halt the Procedure:	Cease the aesthetic treatment immediately to prevent further injection or surgical trauma that may exacerbate the vascular compromise.
Inform the Patient:	Communicate with the patient transparently about the situation. Explain the need for prompt action and reassure them that steps are being taken to address the issue.
Positioning:	Place the patient in an elevated position to optimize blood flow to the affected area. This can help reduce swelling and alleviate vascular compromise.
Warm compresses:	Apply warm compresses to the affected area. Heat can help dilate blood vessels and improve blood flow. However, avoid excessive heat to prevent burns.
Administration of Hyaluronidase:	If the vascular compromise is related to dermal filler injections, the prompt administration of Hyaluronidase can dissolve the filler material and restore blood flow. This should be performed under the supervision of a qualified healthcare professional.
Emergency Consultation:	Seek immediate consultation with a vascular surgeon or other relevant specialists to assess the severity of the situation and determine further interventions.
Monitoring:	Continuously monitor the patient's vital signs, assess the affected area for changes, and document the progression or resolution of symptoms.

With regards emergency Measures and Interventions to Mitigate Vascular Compromise below steps should be considered [5, 7, 8, 11]. A recent study by Goodman et al [14], states that the use of aspiration is considered limiting, and that other preventative measures such as continuous movement when injecting, slow injection speed, low extrusion force and small volumes, in conjunction with an in-depth understanding of the safer injection planes pertaining to vascular anatomy, may mitigate intravascular incidents [14].

Emergency Measures to Mitigate Vascular Compromise

Aspiration and Injection Technique:	• If applicable, aspirate before injection to avoid intravascular injection. Implement slow injection techniques to minimize the risk of vascular compromise.
Topical Nitroglycerin:	• In some cases, topical nitroglycerin can be applied to enhance blood flow and relieve vasospasm. This should be done under medical supervision.
Oxygen Therapy:	• Administer supplemental oxygen to improve tissue oxygenation. Adequate oxygen supply is crucial for mitigating the effects of vascular compromise.
Anticoagulant Therapy:	• In consultation with a specialist, anticoagulant therapy may be considered to prevent clot formation and enhance blood flow.
Hyperbaric Oxygen Therapy (HBOT):	• In severe cases, HBOT may be recommended. It involves breathing pure oxygen in a pressurized room and can aid in tissue oxygenation and healing

5.1.4 Best Practice for Safe Facial Aesthetic Treatment

Establishing and adhering to recommended guidelines and protocols is crucial for ensuring the safe and effective practice of facial aesthetic procedures and preventing vascular complications. Here are comprehensive guidelines to minimize the risk of vascular compromise:

In the preparation for facial aesthetic procedures, several key considerations and practices are essential for ensuring patient safety and optimal outcomes.

Before any procedure, a thorough pre-procedural assessment is important. This involves a comprehensive review of the patient's medical history, with a particular focus on vascular conditions, allergies, and any prior complications. Additionally, practitioners should engage in open discussions with patients to understand their expectations and provide a realistic overview of the anticipated outcomes. During the informed consent process, potential risks, especially those related to vascular complications, should be clearly communicated. Patients should be educated about the signs and symptoms of complications and when to seek immediate medical attention [1, 5, 8, 9, 11].

Practitioners must possess the necessary expertise to perform facial aesthetic procedures safely. This involves undergoing comprehensive training in facial anatomy, injection techniques, and the recognition of potential complications. Continuous education is crucial to staying abreast of the latest advancements and safety measures in the field. Certification in specific procedures, meeting the standards established by relevant medical boards or associations, is essential to ensure practitioners' competency and adherence to recognized standards [1, 5, 7].

Executing the procedure itself demands a high level of skill and understanding. Practitioners should possess a profound knowledge of facial vascular anatomy, identifying arteries, veins, and potential anastomoses. Careful consideration should be given to injection sites, avoiding high-risk areas such as the glabella and nose. Techniques to minimize the risk of vascular compromise include aspiration before injection to check for blood return, thus avoiding intravascular injection. Additionally, utilizing slow and controlled injection techniques is imperative in mitigating the risk of complications. For the advanced injector with a thorough understanding of the physics of colour Doppler, use of ultrasound utilising colour Doppler mode to perform the injection of filler in real time would potentially be the most effective way to avoid or minimise an inadvertent arterial or venous injection (refer to Videos 5.1 and 5.2).

Being prepared for potential emergencies is a fundamental aspect of responsible practice. Emergency equipment, including hyaluronidase, nitroglycerin cream, and oxygen administration supplies, should be readily available. Practitioners need to be trained to immediately recognize signs of vascular compromise and have a clear protocol for initiating emergency measures. This includes actions such as applying warm compresses, administering hyaluronidase, and promptly notifying relevant specialists.

The responsibility extends into the post-procedural phase. Patients should be monitored for an appropriate duration to detect any signs of complications. Clear post-procedure instructions, along with emergency contact information, should be provided to patients. Follow-up appointments should be scheduled to assess the outcomes of the procedure, address any concerns, and manage complications if they arise.

Maintaining detailed records of each procedure is essential for accountability and continuous improvement. This includes documenting the type and volume of products used, injection sites, and any adverse events. Encouraging peer reviews and case discussions facilitates shared learning from experiences and complications. Regular updates to protocols, informed by emerging evidence and collective experiences, contribute to a dynamic and evolving approach to patient care and safety in facial aesthetic procedures.

By implementing these guidelines and protocols, practitioners can significantly reduce the risk of vascular complications during facial aesthetic procedures, promoting patient safety and achieving optimal outcomes. Regular training, staying informed about the latest developments, and fostering a culture of continuous improvement are integral components of a safe and effective aesthetic practice [3, 5, 7, 8, 11].

5.2 Soft Tissue Infections

In the realm of facial aesthetic procedures, soft tissue infections can involve various microbial pathogens. Bacterial culprits commonly include Staphylococcus aureus, notorious for causing cellulitis and abscesses, and different Streptococcus species, particularly Group A Streptococcus (GAS), contributing to conditions like cellulitis and erysipelas. Anaerobic bacteria, such as Bacteroides and Prevotella species, may also be implicated, often associated with infections related to dental procedures. Viral pathogens, like the Herpes Simplex Virus (HSV) with its potential for reactivation leading to herpetic lesions, and Human Papillomavirus (HPV), known for wart-like lesions, add to the infectious spectrum. Fungal infections, typically involving Candida species, become noteworthy, especially in immunocompromised individuals [2, 5, 7, 8, 15, 16].

The transmission of these pathogens can occur through various routes, including direct contact with contaminated surfaces, instruments, or hands, as well as airborne transmission through respiratory droplets. Hematogenous spread, wherein bloodborne pathogens enter the bloodstream during facial procedures, poses an additional risk. Predisposing factors amplify the susceptibility to soft tissue infections, encompassing poor hygiene practices, immunosuppression, disruption of the skin barrier during procedures, and pre-existing skin conditions like eczema [1].

Each pathogen has distinct microbiological characteristics and clinical implications. Staphylococcus aureus, a gram-positive coccus that may be methicillin-resistant (MRSA), is associated with cellulitis, abscesses, and potential systemic infections. Streptococcus species, also gram-positive cocci, particularly Group A Streptococcus, can lead to rapidly progressing cellulitis or erysipelas. Anaerobic bacteria, represented by Bacteroides, Prevotella, and Fusobacterium species, are often involved in infections following dental procedures, resulting in abscess formation. Viral pathogens like HSV, a double-stranded DNA virus, can cause reactivation and painful vesicular eruptions, while Candida species, yeasts commonly represented by Candida albicans, may cause localized or systemic fungal infections, especially in immunocompromised individuals [1].

Understanding these microbiological characteristics and clinical implications is paramount in preventing and managing soft tissue infections in facial aesthetic procedures. Practitioners must prioritize infection control measures, adhere to sterile techniques, and consider predisposing factors to minimize the risk of post-procedural infections. Regular education and training in infection prevention protocols are essential for maintaining patient safety in the aesthetic practice.

5.2.1 Clinical Presentation and Diagnosis of Soft Tissue Infections Post-Aesthetic Treatment

Post-facial aesthetic procedures, soft tissue infections can manifest in diverse clinical presentations. These manifestations may include localized symptoms such as redness, swelling, and pain, extending to more severe signs such as cellulitis, abscess formation, or, in extreme cases, systemic symptoms like fever and malaise. The specific clinical manifestations can vary based on the type of pathogen involved, the extent of infection, and the patient's overall health. For instance, bacterial infections may present with rapidly spreading erythema and tenderness, while viral infections might manifest as vesicular lesions. Fungal infections may exhibit a range of symptoms from localized irritation to more severe tissue involvement [2, 5, 7, 8, 15, 16].

Accurate diagnosis of soft tissue infections following facial aesthetic procedures is pivotal for effective management (Fig. 5.3). Diagnostic

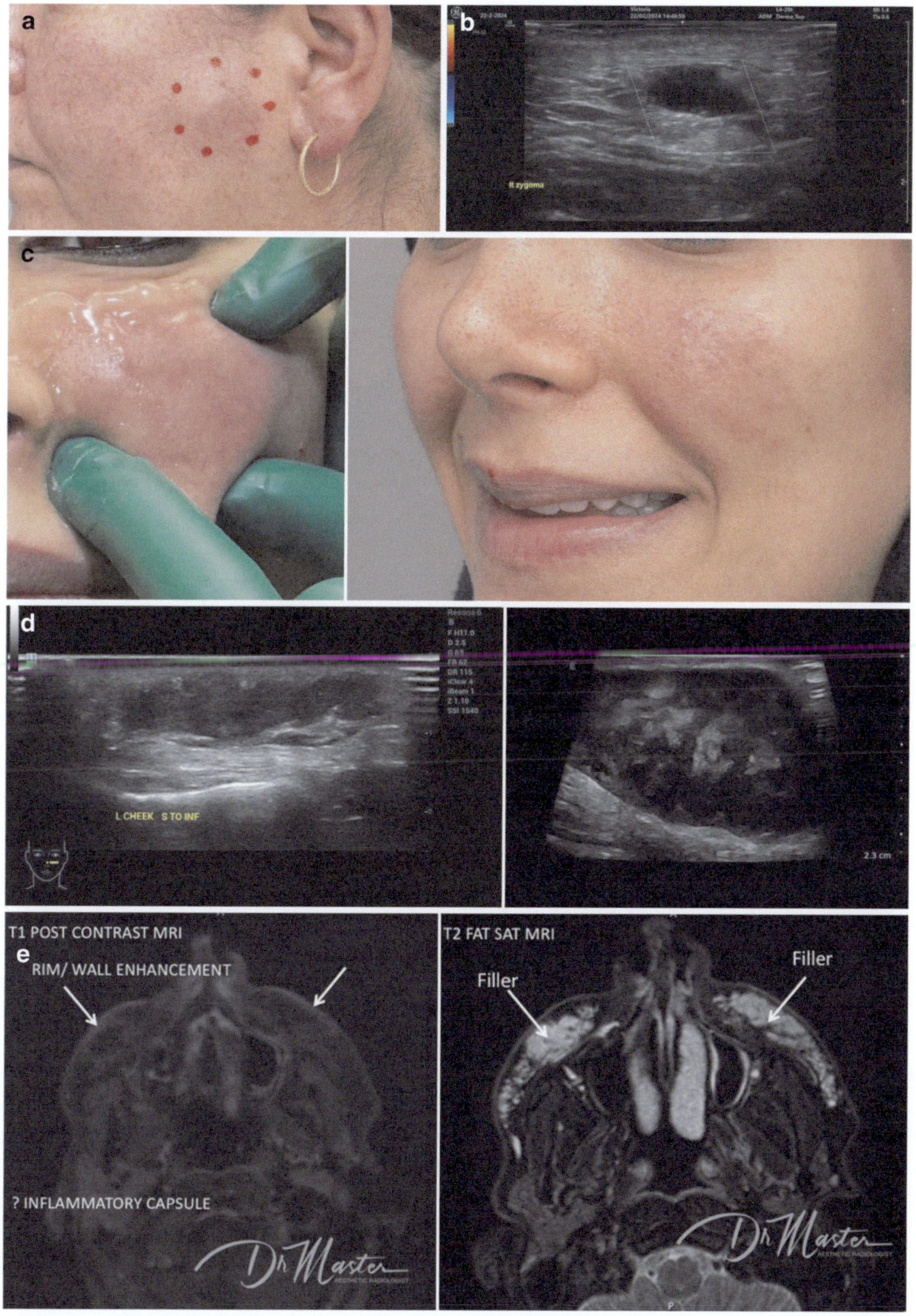

Fig. 5.3 Clinical and ultrasound images of a sterile abscess (Case study 3)
(**a**) Patient presented with a fluctuant, erythematous, localized painful nodule, 3 months post filler injection (hyaluronic acid) (**b**) in the pre auricular region, inferior to the zygomatic bone, a localized hardened nodule, 0.7 ml was aspirated and sent for Culture (MC&S). Report found polymorphs present, however negative culture indicated
Patient was treated with 3 ml saline, 2 ml Xylocaine 2 % and 3000 IU Hyaluronidase. Special thanks to Dr Peter Callen

criteria often include a thorough clinical examination, considering the patient's symptoms, physical findings, and relevant medical history. Investigative methods encompass laboratory tests such as complete blood count (CBC), cultures, and imaging studies like ultrasound or magnetic resonance imaging (MRI). Blood cultures can help identify systemic involvement, while tissue cultures may be crucial for pinpointing the causative pathogen. Additionally, imaging can aid in assessing the extent of infection and guiding appropriate interventions [1, 5, 7, 8, 16–21].

5.2.2 Management of Soft Tissue Infections in Facial Aesthetics

Soft tissue infections following facial aesthetic treatments require a comprehensive approach involving both medical and surgical interventions. In milder cases, antimicrobial therapy plays a crucial role. Initial empirical treatment often includes broad-spectrum antibiotics, targeting common pathogens associated with soft tissue infections. Culture and sensitivity testing should guide subsequent antibiotic choices for more targeted therapy. In cases of abscess formation or severe infections, surgical interventions such as incision and drainage (I&D) may be necessary to remove purulent material and alleviate pressure. Surgical debridement becomes essential in cases of necrotizing infections to remove necrotic tissue and prevent further spread. The choice between medical and surgical interventions depends on the severity of the infection, the involvement of deeper tissues, and the response to initial treatments.

A comprehensive protocol for managing soft tissue infections involves a step-by-step guide for the appropriate use of antimicrobial agents, drainage procedures, and wound care. The protocol recommends initiating empirical antibiotic therapy based on the suspected pathogens and infection severity. Before starting antibiotics, collecting appropriate specimens for culture is essential to adjust the regimen based on culture results. The route of administration should be tailored to the infection severity, with intravenous therapy for severe cases transitioning to oral agents as the patient improves. Antibiotics should be administered for an appropriate duration guided by the resolution of clinical symptoms and normalization of laboratory parameters [5, 7, 8, 11].

Regarding drainage procedures, practitioners are advised to consider incision and drainage (I&D) for abscess formation, purulent collections, or cases where the response to antibiotics alone is insufficient. Aseptic techniques should be employed during drainage procedures to minimize the risk of secondary infection. In evolving infections, repeat drainage procedures may be necessary to ensure the complete removal of infected material.

In terms of wound care, the protocol emphasizes regular cleaning with mild antiseptics to prevent secondary infections. Appropriate dressing changes should be implemented to maintain a sterile environment and support optimal wound healing. Practitioners are encouraged to actively monitor the wound for signs of healing, including reduced erythema, swelling, and pain.

This comprehensive protocol ensures a systematic and evidence-based approach to managing soft tissue infections, aiming to optimize patient outcomes, minimize complications, and uphold effective and ethical clinical practice.

Soft tissue infections in the context of facial aesthetic procedures may give rise to various complications and long-term sequelae. Complications include the formation of disfiguring scars, persistent erythema, and pigmentation changes. Severe infections, if not promptly and adequately managed, may lead to tissue necrosis and deformities. Systemic complications, although rare, can occur, necessitating vigilant monitoring and intervention. Long-term sequelae may involve psychological effects, such as patient dissatisfaction, anxiety, or reluctance to undergo future aesthetic procedures. In cases of extensive soft tissue damage, reconstructive surgeries may be required to restore both form and function [1, 8].

The management of soft tissue infections following facial aesthetic treatments necessitates a tailored approach, combining medical and surgical interventions. A step-by-step guide to antimicrobial use, drainage procedures, and wound care is essential for optimal outcomes. Recognizing potential complications and understanding long-term sequelae is crucial for comprehensive patient care in the aftermath of facial aesthetic procedures.

5.2.3 Prevention of Soft Tissue Infections in Facial Aesthetic Procedures

Preventing soft tissue infections following facial aesthetic treatments requires a thorough analysis of preventive strategies and infection control measures. Firstly, meticulous adherence to hygiene practices is paramount. Practitioners should implement strict hand hygiene protocols, ensuring hands are thoroughly washed and disinfected before and after each procedure. Sterilization of instruments and equipment, including needles, syringes, and surgical tools, is critical to prevent contamination. Furthermore, the use of disposable materials and single-use items wherever possible can significantly reduce the risk of microbial transmission. Regular cleaning and disinfection of the treatment environment, including surfaces and furniture, contribute to maintaining asepsis [1].

Sterile techniques, thorough pre-procedural assessments, and meticulous post-treatment care play pivotal roles in preventing soft tissue infections. The utilization of sterile draping, gloves, and gowns during procedures creates a barrier against potential pathogens. Pre-procedural assessments involve a comprehensive examination of the patient's medical history, assessing potential risk factors, and ensuring that the patient is in optimal health for the planned procedure. Post-treatment care includes diligent wound management, emphasizing proper dressing changes and monitoring for any signs of infection. Clear communication with patients about post-treatment care instructions is essential to encourage adherence and prompt reporting of any concerns.

Establishing and following recommended guidelines and protocols are essential for maintaining asepsis and minimizing the incidence of soft tissue infections in facial aesthetic procedures. These guidelines should encompass:

The preparation for facial aesthetic procedures involves a systematic approach encompassing several key steps to ensure both the safety of the patient and the efficacy of the procedure.

To establish a foundation for aseptic conditions, the treatment area must be thoroughly disinfected. This includes meticulous cleaning to eliminate potential pathogens. Additionally, the availability of sterile instruments and disposables is essential, ensuring that all equipment used during the procedure is free from contamination. Stringent adherence to appropriate hygiene practices is a prerequisite, involving not only the disinfection of the treatment area but also the conscientious handwashing and use of personal protective equipment by all practitioners involved in the procedure.

Conducting a comprehensive pre-procedural assessment is integral to identify any contraindications or risk factors for infection that may affect the patient's suitability for the procedure. This involves a thorough examination of the patient's medical history and overall health. Equally important is the transparent communication of potential risks during the informed consent process. Patients must be well-informed about the nature of the procedure, potential complications, and the importance of their role in adherence to post-treatment care.

Maintaining sterile conditions during the actual procedure is critical to prevent infections. Aseptic techniques, involving the use of sterile drapes, gloves, and the establishment of a sterile field, are essential during injections, surgeries, or any procedure involving skin penetration. The application of these techniques minimizes the risk of contamination and upholds the integrity of the treatment environment. Implementing strict sterilization protocols for reusable instruments and equipment is a fundamental aspect of infection control. This involves adhering to industry standards and guidelines for the sterilization process. Regular monitoring and validation of sterilization equipment are essential to ensure its efficacy and the consistent production of sterile instruments for each procedure.

The responsibility for infection prevention extends into the post-treatment phase. Providing patients with clear and detailed post-treatment care instructions is crucial. Emphasis should be placed on wound care practices, medication adherence, and the prompt reporting of any complications. Scheduled follow-up appointments facilitate ongoing monitoring of the healing process and provide opportunities to address any emerging concerns or complications promptly. Practitioners involved in facial aesthetic procedures should be committed to continuous learning and professional development. Regular updates on the latest infection control measures, aseptic techniques, and guidelines are imperative. This commitment to ongoing education ensures that practitioners remain well-informed and proficient in implementing the latest advancements in the field, contributing to the maintenance of high standards of patient care and safety [5, 7, 8, 11].

5.2.4 Legal and Ethical Considerations in the Management of Complications in Facial Aesthetics

Complications arising from facial aesthetic treatments, notably vascular compromise, and soft tissue infections, carry significant legal and ethical implications. In the legal realm, practitioners may be subject to litigation if complications lead to adverse outcomes. Establishing negligence requires scrutiny of the practitioner's adherence to standard care practices, adequate training, and the fulfillment of legal duties. Ethically, the principle of beneficence, prioritizing the well-being of the patient, is paramount. Practitioners must ensure that procedures are performed with the highest standards of care, and any complications are promptly addressed to minimize harm and uphold patient safety.

In the context of managing complications in facial aesthetics, the patient's rights, informed consent, and professional obligations become central considerations. Patients have the right to expect a standard of care that prioritizes their safety and well-being. Should complications arise, patients retain the right to be informed, involved in decision-making, and to receive appropriate follow-up care. Respect for patient autonomy is crucial, necessitating transparent communication about potential risks and complications associated with the procedures. Informed consent is not only a legal requirement but a fundamental ethical principle. Practitioners have an obligation to provide comprehensive information about the risks and benefits of the proposed procedures. This includes the potential for complications such as vascular compromise and soft tissue infections. Informed consent empowers the patient to make autonomous decisions and fosters trust between the practitioner and patient. If complications do occur, the documentation of a thorough informed consent process becomes a critical defense against potential legal challenges [1].

Practitioners in facial aesthetics have ethical and professional obligations to prioritize patient safety and well-being. This encompasses maintaining competence through ongoing education, staying informed about the latest developments in the field, and ensuring that procedures are performed within the scope of their expertise. When complications arise, practitioners have a duty to promptly recognize, disclose, and manage these complications. Timely and appropriate intervention can mitigate harm and minimize the potential legal consequences. Balancing legal and ethical considerations involves a delicate interplay between protecting the practitioner's professional reputation and upholding patient rights. Striking this balance requires adherence to ethical principles, ensuring that patients are treated with respect and dignity, and their rights to autonomy and informed decision-making are upheld. At the same time, practitioners must navigate the legal landscape by documenting thorough informed consent processes, maintaining detailed records, and seeking legal advice if complications lead to disputes.

In conclusion, the legal and ethical implications of complications in facial aesthetics, particularly vascular compromise, and soft tissue infections, demand a meticulous approach from practitioners. Adherence to ethical principles, upholding patient rights, obtaining informed consent, and fulfilling professional obligations are pivotal in mitigating legal risks and, more importantly, in ensuring the well-being of the patients undergoing facial aesthetic treatments.

References

1. Rayess HM, Svider PF, Hanba C, Patel VS, DeJoseph LM, Carron M, et al. A cross-sectional analysis of adverse events and litigation for injectable fillers. JAMA Facial Plast Surg. 2018;20(3):207–14. https://doi.org/10.1001/jamafacial.2017.1888.
2. Beleznay K, Humphries S, Carruthers JDA, Carruthers A. Vascular compromise from soft tissue augmentation: experience with 12 cases and recommendations for optimal outcomes. J Clin Aesthet Dermatol. 2014;7(9):37–43.
3. Goodman GJ, Roberts S, Callan P. Experience and Management of Intravascular Injection with facial fillers: results of a multinational survey of experienced injectors. Aesth Plast Surg. 2016;40(4):549–55. https://doi.org/10.1007/s00266-016-0658-1.
4. Beleznay K, Carruthers JD, Humphrey S, Jones D. Avoiding and treating blindness from fillers: a review of the world literature. Dermatologic Surg. 2015;41(10):1097–117. https://doi.org/10.1097/DSS.0000000000000486.
5. Sundaram H, Signorini M, Liew S, Trindade de Almeida AR, Wu Y, Vieira Braz A, et al. Global Aesthetics Consensus: Botulinum Toxin Type A--Evidence-Based Review, Emerging Concepts, and Consensus Recommendations for Aesthetic Use, Including Updates on Complications. Plast Reconstr Surg 2016; 137(3):518e-529e. https://doi.org/10.1097/01.prs.0000475758.63709.23.
6. Samizadeh S, De Boulle K. Complications of toxins and fillers in facial aesthetics. Prim Dent J. 2023;12(3):65–72.
7. Daines SM, Williams EF. Complications associated with injectable soft-tissue fillers: a 5-year retrospective review. JAMA Facial Plast Surg. 2013;15(3):226–31. https://doi.org/10.1001/jamafacial.2013.798.
8. Alam M, Dover JS. Management of complications and sequelae with temporary injectable fillers. Plast Reconstr Surg. 2007;120(6 Suppl):98S–105S. https://doi.org/10.1097/01.prs.0000248859.14788.60.
9. Buchanan PJ, Grossman JAI, Price AE, Reddy C, Chopan M, Chim H. The use of botulinum toxin injection for brachial plexus birth injuries: a systematic review of the literature. Hand (NY). 2019;14(2):150–4. https://doi.org/10.1177/1558944718760038.
10. Sito G, Manzoni V, Sommariva R. Vascular complications after facial filler injection: a literature review and meta-analysis. J Clin Aesth Dermatol. 2019;12(6):E65–72.
11. Hood K, Ganesh Kumar N, Kaoutzanis C, Higdon KK. Hematomas in aesthetic surgery. Aesthet Surg J. 2018;38(9):1013–25. https://doi.org/10.1093/asj/sjx236.
12. Kim SH. Interpretation of peripheral arterial and venous Doppler waveforms: a consensus statement from the Society for Vascular Medicine and Society for vascular ultrasound. Vasc Med. 2020;25(5):484–506.
13. Tucunduva MJ, Tucunduva-Neto R, Saieg M, Costa AL, de Freitas C. Vascular mapping of the face: B-mode and doppler ultrasonography study. Med Oral Patol Oral Cir Bucal. 2016;21(2):e135–41. https://doi.org/10.4317/medoral.20754.
14. Goodman GJ, Magnusson MR, Callan P, Roberts S, Hart S, Lin F, et al. Aspiration before tissue filler-an exercise in futility and unsafe practice. Aesthet Surg J. 2022;42(1):89–101. https://doi.org/10.1093/asj/sjab036.
15. Wu WT, Chang KV, Chang HC, Chen LR, Kuan CH, Kao JT, et al. Ultrasound imaging of the facial muscles and relevance with Botulinum toxin injections: a pictorial essay and narrative review. Toxins (Basel). 2022;14(2) https://doi.org/10.3390/toxins14020101.
16. Beer K. Dermal fillers and combinations of fillers for facial rejuvenation. Dermatol Clin. 2009;27(4):427–32. https://doi.org/10.1016/j.det.2009.08.011.
17. Ryu JH, Shim JH, Yeom JH, Shin WJ, Cho SY, Jeon WJ. Ultrasound-guided greater occipital nerve block with botulinum toxin for patients with chronic headache in the occipital area: a randomized controlled trial. Korean J Anesthesiol. 2019;72(5):479–85. https://doi.org/10.4097/kja.19145.
18. Arlette JP, Trotter MJ. Anatomic location of hyaluronic acid filler material injected into nasolabial fold: a histologic study. Dermatologic Surg. 2008;34(Suppl 1):S56–62. https://doi.org/10.1111/j.1524-4725.2008.34244.x. discussion S-3
19. Ambroziak M, Noszczyk B, Pietruski P, Guz W, Paluch L. Elastography reference values of facial skin elasticity. Postepy Dermatol Alergol. 2019;36(5):626–34. https://doi.org/10.5114/ada.2018.77502.
20. Lee HJ, Jung SJ, Kim ST, Kim HJ. Ultrasonographic considerations for safe and efficient Botulinum neurotoxin injection in Masseteric hypertrophy. Toxins (Basel). 2021;13(1) https://doi.org/10.3390/toxins13010028.
21. Haddock NT, Saadeh PB, Boutros S, Thorne CH. The tear trough and lid/cheek junction: anatomy and implications for surgical correction. Plast Reconstr Surg. 2009;123(4):1332–40. https://doi.org/10.1097/PRS.0b013e31819f2b36.

6 Ultrasound Protocol in Facial Aesthetics

6.1 Lower Face

Each section of the face will be approached using a stepwise approach to sonographic imaging, with easy-to-identify, surface anatomy markers to help discern between key target areas during imaging.

For the lower face, the masseter muscle (Fig. 6.1) serves as the starting point for the ultrasound protocol, as it is easily palpated during dynamic clenching of the jaw, and easily differentiated on ultrasound.

6.1.1 Masseter Muscle

Tips:

The masseter is a landmark muscle easily identifiable.

Measure the masseter muscle in the anterior-posterior plane at rest and during contraction as reference pretreatment with neurotoxin.

Follow up measurement can be done in the same plane and orientation at rest and contracted post treatment with neurotoxin.

The transducer is placed 1 cm superior to the mandibular body in the transverse plane at the midpoint between the mentum and mandibular angle. One may need to slide the transducer posteriorly to visualize the entire masseter muscle depending on the size of the masseter and the probe being utilized. Confirm the presence of the masseter muscle through clenching of teeth during dynamic sonographic imaging in the transverse plane identify the superficial head of masseter and place at center of the image. Fig. 6.2) Start at point 1	Fig. 6.2 Transverse sonographic image of the masseter muscle
Split screen to demonstrate masseter muscle at rest on Screen 1 and during contraction on Screen 2 Fig. 6.3 Annotate above screens as neutral/at rest and contracted.	Fig. 6.3 Split screen view of the masseter muscle
Use dynamic imaging to assess the superficial, intermediate and deep muscle bellies. Take note of the three variants of the masseter muscle bellies seen on ultrasound (Fig. 6.4). Type A—The deep internal tendon lies in the anterior thirds of the muscle belly, between the superficial and deep muscle groups. Type B—The deep internal tendon lies within the posterior third of the muscle belly, between the superficial and deep muscle groups. Type C—The deep internal tendon covers predominantly the most inferior part of the masseter muscle.	Fig. 6.4 Three variants of the masseter muscle

K. Malherbe, S. Roberts, *Ultrasound Protocol for Facial Aesthetics*,
https://doi.org/10.1007/978-3-031-75949-9_6

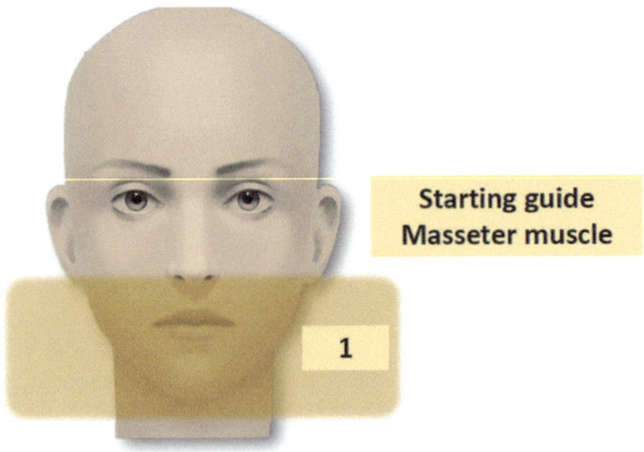

Fig. 6.1 Sonographic stepwise approach for the lower face
Start at point 1 for imaging of the lower face. The masseter muscle remains the starting point to reach all the other lower face muscles

Fig. 6.2 Transverse image of the masseter muscle
Placing the transducer in transverse orientation will demonstrate the masseter muscle

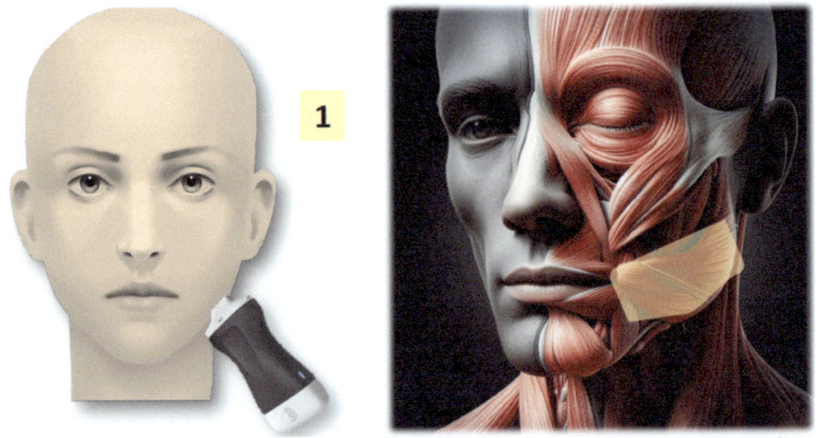

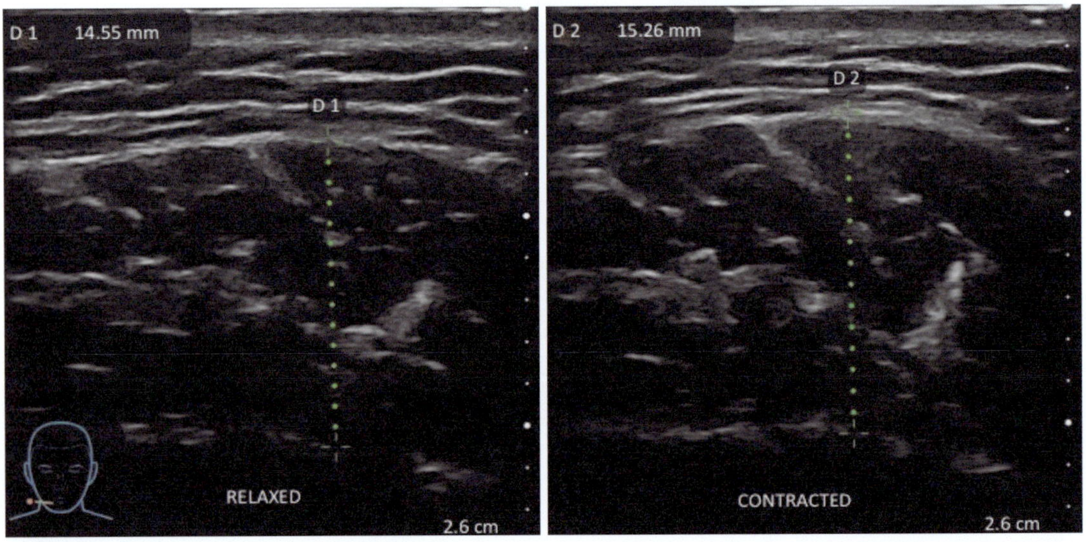

Fig. 6.3 Split screen view of the bilateral masseter muscles demonstrating reduced width of muscle during relaxed phase in comparison to contraction of muscle

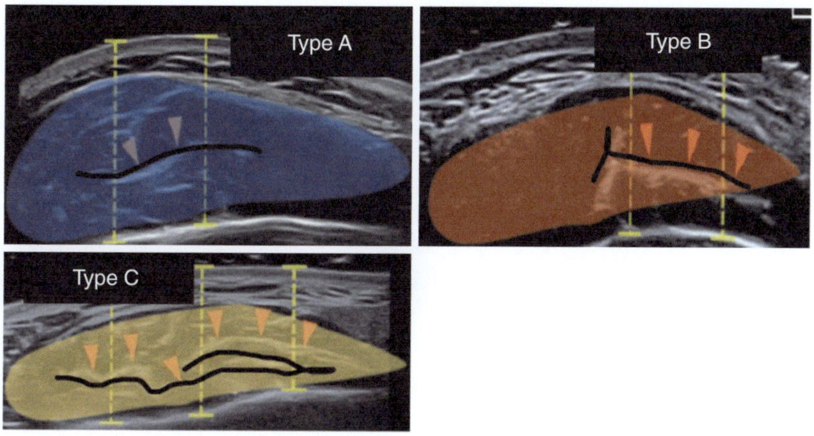

Fig. 6.4 The three variants of the masseter muscle
Three variants are known of the masseter muscle relating to the deep internal tendon (DIT)
Image A: DIT extends within the midregion of the muscle belly
Image B: DIT extends towards from mid to the anterior border of the muscle belly
Image C: DIT extends across the entire anterior and posterior borders of the muscle belly with multiple myotendinous fibrous divisions (indicated by orange arrow heads)

6.1.2 Parotid Gland

Tips:
Assess proximity of the parotid gland to the masseter muscle
The parotid gland has a diffuse hyperechoic appearance on ultrasound.
The masseter and parotid gland may be injected with neurotoxin for facial reshaping.
Lymph nodes may be identified in the planned region of interest through use of Color Doppler

Place the transducer in transverse orientation, the midpoint of the transducer surface is aligned with the anterior border of the masseter muscle. Glide the transducer in the same anatomical plane in a posterior direction towards the External Acoustic Meatus (EAM) (Fig. 6.5). The first hyperechoic structure identified just posterior to the masseter muscle is the parotid gland. **Move from point 1 to point 2.**	Fig. 6.5 Parotid gland in relation to the masseter muscle
Assess presence of any lymphadenopathy in the region of interest planned for filler enhancement.(Fig. 6.6)	Fig. 6.6 Parotid gland and lymphadenopathy

6.1.3 Facial Artery and Vein

Tips:
Important landmark to assess before and after treatment to assess proximity of vessels to the area of interest to avoid vascular occlusion when injecting fillers.
Arteries are tortuous and pulsatile.
Veins tend to be larger compared to arteries and are compressible.

Transducer in transverse orientation. Midpoint of transducer surface on the anterior border of the masseter muscle. In the same anatomical plane, glide the transducer in an anterior direction towards the oral commissure. The anterior portion of the masseter muscle should remain in the image (as seen in Fig. 6.7.) **Move from point 1 to point 3**	Fig. 6.7 Transverse view of the facial artery
Color Doppler mode should be activated, with the color box placed just along the anterior border of the masseter muscle to demonstrate the facial vein and artery in cross sectional orientation. The colour box may need to be steered to detect the vessels. Power Doppler may be used to detect vessels. (Fig. 6.8)	Fig. 6.8 Color Doppler and the facial artery
The facial vein lies posterior to the facial artery at this point. (Fig. 6.9)	Fig. 6.9 Sonographic view of the facial vein

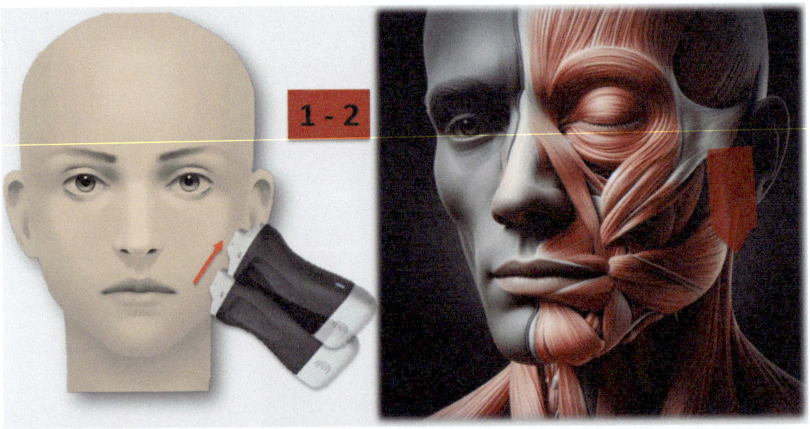

Fig. 6.5 Parotid gland in relation to the masseter muscle Move from point 1 (masseter muscle) to point two, by gliding the probe posterior towards the external acoustic meatus

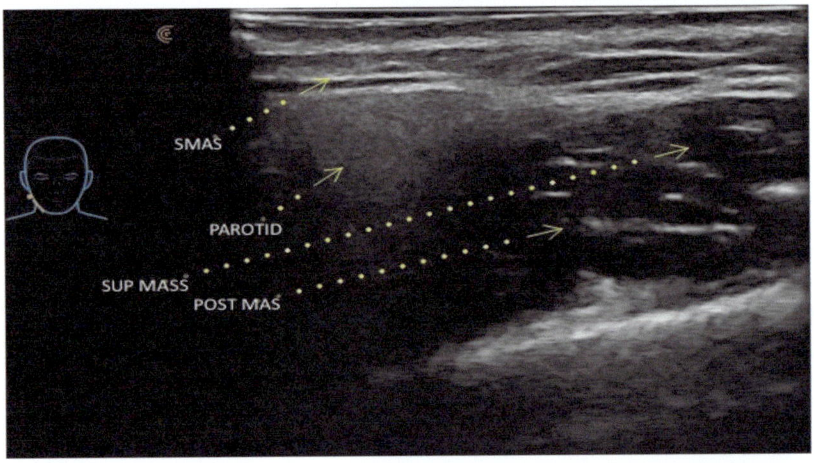

Fig. 6.6 Parotid gland and associated lymphadenopathy Indicating the various layers associated with the parotid gland just posterior to the masseter muscle belly

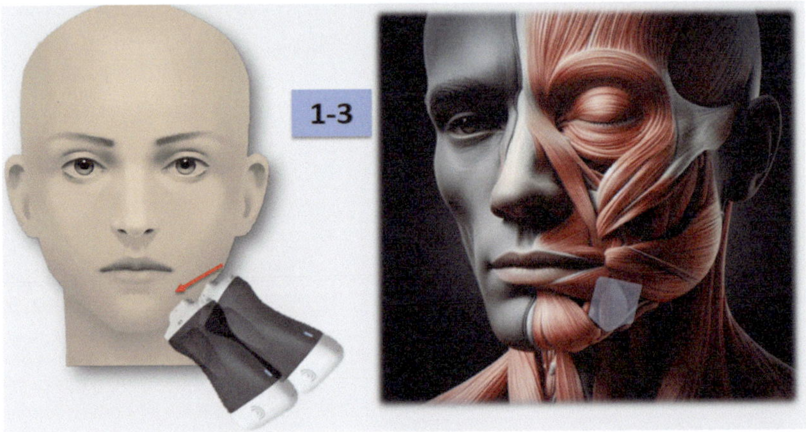

Fig. 6.7 Transverse view of the facial artery Move from point 1 (masseter to point 3, by gliding the probe anterior to the masseter muscle

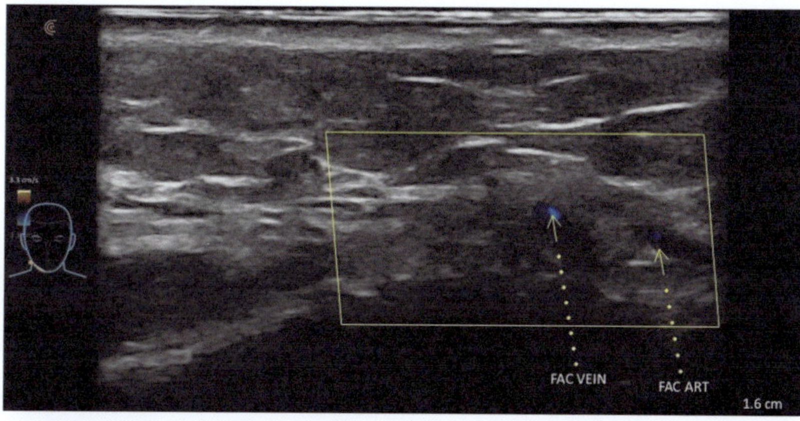

Fig. 6.8 Color Doppler and the facial artery The vessel visualised closest to the masseter muscle belly is the facial vein, thereafter the facial artery is visualised

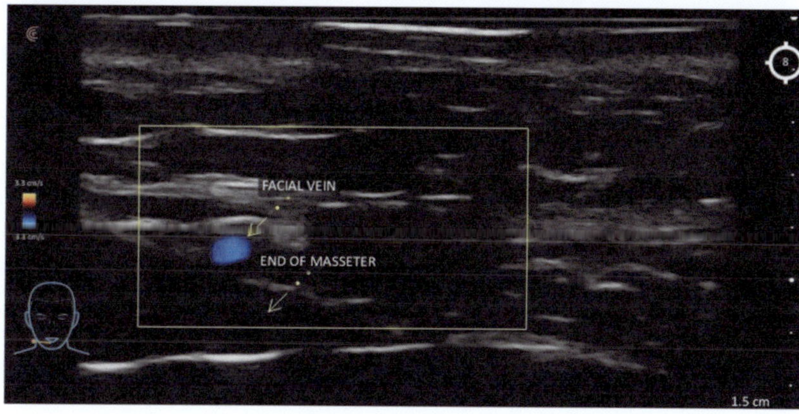

Fig. 6.9 Sonographic view of the facial vein Just anterior to the masseter muscle, the facial vein is demonstrated in this figure in transverse plane

6.1.4 Risorius Muscle

Tips:

Difficult muscle to visualize on ultrasound.

Locating risorius on ultrasound may help prevent inadvertent injection of neurotoxin into risorius when injecting the masseter muscle as this may result in shortening of the patient's smile.

Transducer in transverse orientation with the midpoint of the transducer along the anterior border of the masseter, a systematic inferior to superior sweep is performed from the mandibular body upwards towards the maxilla. When present, risorius is a thin, hypoechoic band noted between the anterior border of the masseter and the posterior fibers of the depressor anguli oris muscle Fig. 6.10). Risorius extends from the anterior border of the masseter muscle and is the more superficial band (closest to the skin surface). **Move from point 1 to point 4**	Fig. 6.10 Transverse view of the risorius muscle
The masseter and depressor anguli oris are visualized in the transverse plane. The risorius muscle is visualized in its length as a thin band between the masseter muscle (Fig. 6.11) and the DAO.	Fig. 6.11 Risorius muscle in relation to masseter muscle
Alternate method: Glide the transducer in the transverse plane with the midpoint of the transducer at the anterior border of the masseter muscle. The transducer is then glided superior until two thin hypoechoic bands are noted extending from the masseter muscle belly with bilateral hyperechoic fascia parallel to their course (Fig. 6.12). The more superior band (closest to the skin surface) is the risorius muscle.	Fig. 6.12 Alternate method to visualize risorius muscle on ultrasound
Dynamic imaging of the risorius muscle during lateral pulling of the mouth with the patient smiling, would also result in noting the dynamic pulling action of risorius between DAO and masseter towards a posterior direction. Note in image the difference in distance between contraction and neutral imaging of the risorius in Fig. 6.13.	Fig. 6.13 Dynamic imaging of the risorius muscle

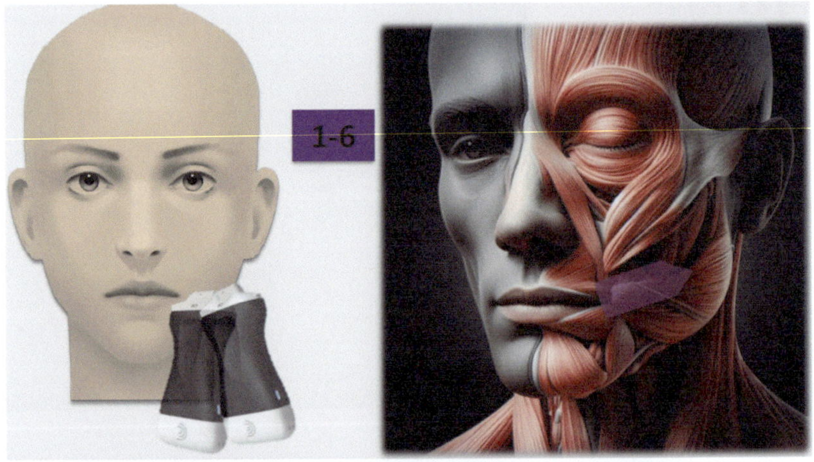

Fig. 6.10 Transverse view of the risorius muscle
Move from point 1 (masseter muscle) to point 6, which is slight superior gliding of the probe to the upper most end of the masseter muscle to visualize a thin hypoechoic band, namely the risorius muscle

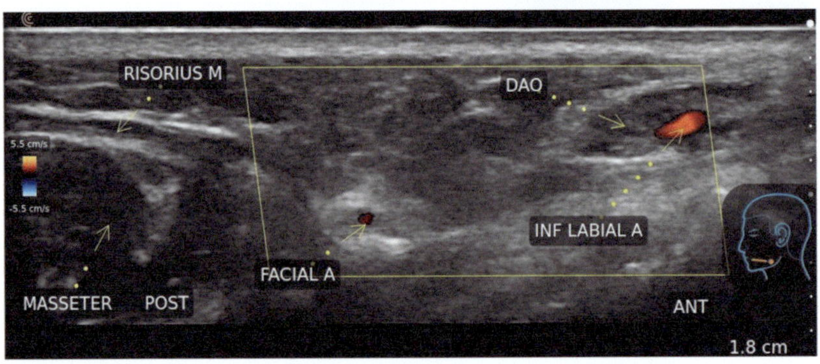

Fig. 6.11 Risorius muscle in relation to the masseter muscle
Using the stepwise approach, moving the probe, in transverse plane, anterior and superior, the first superficial band noted is the risorius muscle. For further confirmation of the muscle belly, animation of the risorius muscle function is used to affirm presence of risorius muscle

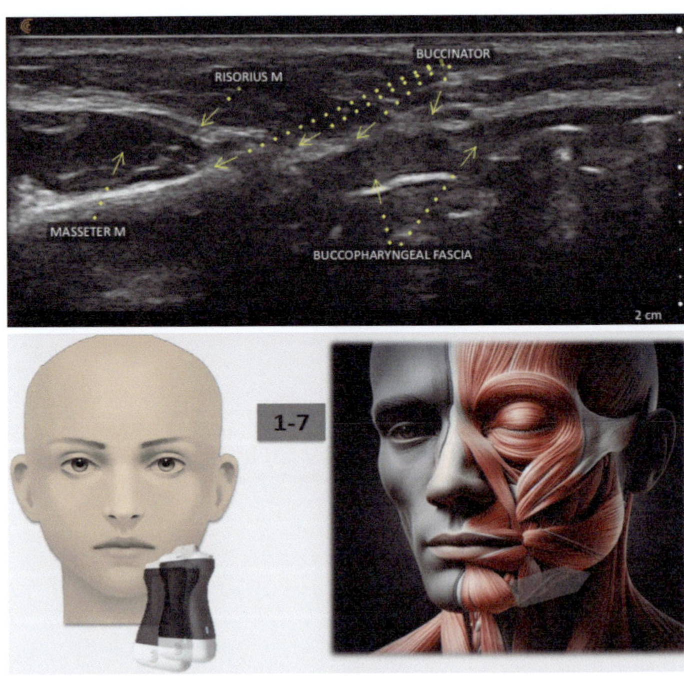

Fig. 6.12 Alternate method to visualize risorius muscle on ultrasound
Alternate method to visualize risorious is to start at Point 1 (masseter) and to move anterior towards the mentum so that both the buccinator and risorius muscle is visualised in relation to the masseter muscle and buccopharyneal fascia

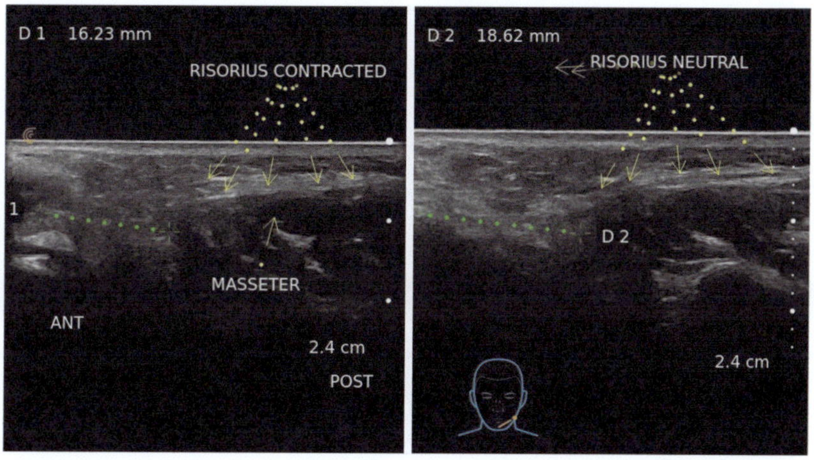

Fig. 6.13 Dynamic imaging of the risorius muscle on ultrasound

6.1.5 Depressor Anguli Oris (DAO) Muscle

Tips:

The DAO is a landmark muscle in the lower face, easily identifiable.

Muscle can be assessed dynamically during sonographic imaging through downwards pulling motion of the lateral commissures of the mouth.

Common target muscle for neuromodulator treatment

Transducer in transverse orientation, the midpoint of the transducer surface starts on the anterior border of the masseter muscle, approximately 1 cm superior to the mandible. Glide transducer in the same anatomical plane more anteriorly. The first muscle belly identified in close relation to the masseter muscle is the DAO (Fig. 6.14). **Move from point 1 to point 5**	Fig. 6.14 Transverse view of DAO
The DAO muscle is assessed in its transverse plane. Deep and more medial to the DAO, is the depressor labii inferioris (DLI) muscle. (Fig. 6.15)	Fig. 6.15 DAO in relation to DLI
DLI—is the thinner hypoechoic muscle belly medial and deep to the DAO DAO—Is the thicker diamond shaped muscle (also known as triangularis) more lateral and closer to masseter muscle than DLI	Fig. 6.16 Oblique sonographic view of DAO
DAO can be visualized with the transducer in an oblique direction. Place heel of transducer lateral to oral commissure on modiolus. Place the toe of the transducer in a longitudinal plane. Sweep the toe of the transducer laterally in an oblique direction to locate DAO from insertion to it's origin. (Fig. 6.16)	
An anatomical landmark to use to demarcate DAO from DLI is the inferior labial artery which lies deep to the DAO but superficial to the DLI Placing the transducer in the transverse plane with the toe of the transducer at the midpoint of the chin. Add a colour Doppler box including the DAO muscle in the box and increase the color gain to visualize the inferior labial artery in the cross section. Glide the transducer in this position from inferior to superior until the inferior labial artery is visualized (Fig. 6.17). The muscle noted just medial to the inferior labial artery, will be the DLI muscle (indicated with red circle)	Fig. 6.17 DAO and the inferior labial artery

6.1.6 Depressor Labii Inferioris (DLI) Muscle

Tips:

Typically, smaller compared to the DAO.

Found deep to and medial to the DAO.

Overactivation of the depressor labii inferioris muscle may cause a droopy appearance of the lower lip, this may be uni- or bilateral, resulting in an asymmetrical smile if unilateral overactivation is noted.

Transducer in transverse orientation with the midpoint of the transducer on the midline of the chin, approximately 1 cm superior to the mandibular body. Glide the transducer in a posterior direction, until only the lateral edge of the mentalis muscle is in the field of view, the next muscle noted superficial to the lateral (Fig. 6.18). **Same position 5 as Depressor anguli oris, the muscle deep to DAO, is the depressor labii inferioris muscle.**	Fig. 6.18 DLI on ultrasound
Transverse orientation of DLI deep to DAO laterally and superficial to mentalis muscle medially (Fig. 6.19)	Fig. 6.19 DLI in relation to DAO and mentalis muscle

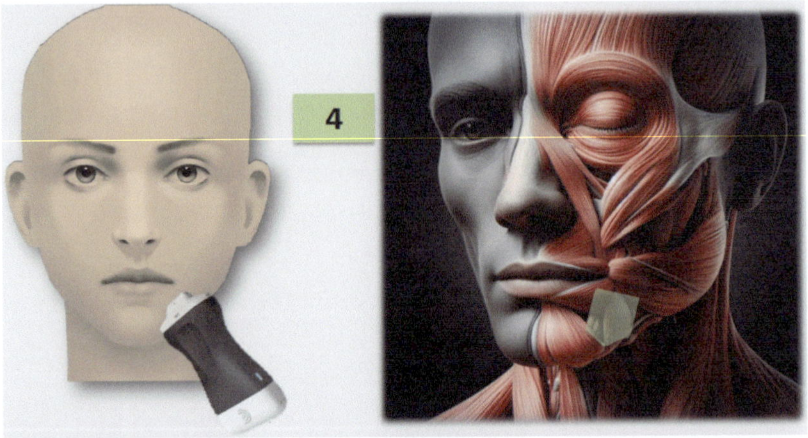

Fig. 6.14 Transverse view of the Depressor Anguli Oris muscle Move from point 1 to point 4, which is 2 cm anterior to the masseter muscle

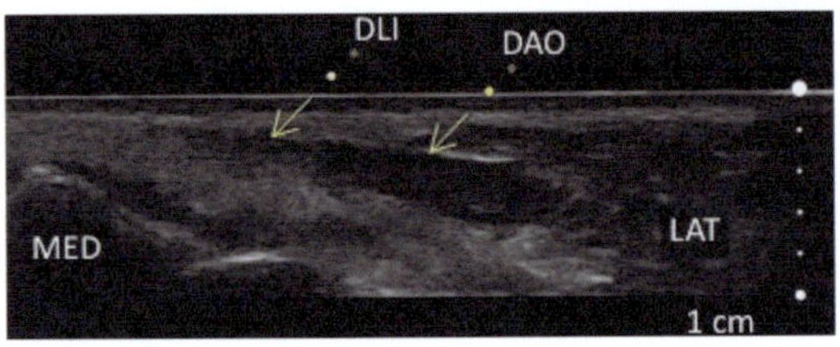

Fig. 6.15 Depressor Anguli Oris muscle in relation to Depressor Labii Inferioris muscle

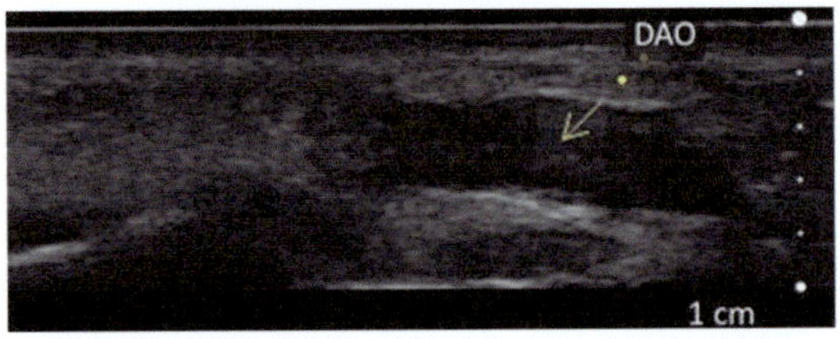

Fig. 6.16 Oblique sonographic view of the Depressor Anguli Oris muscle

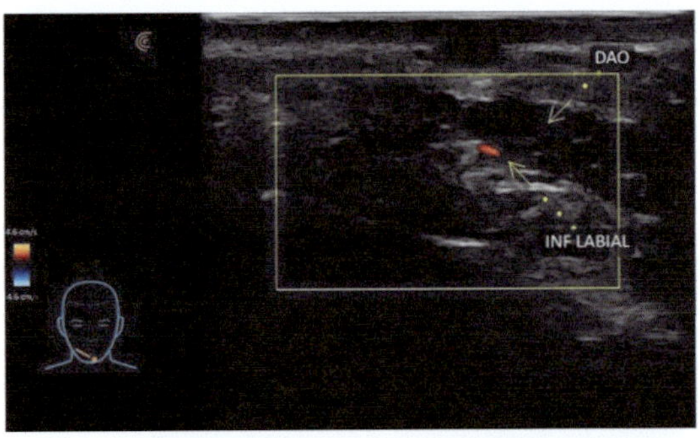

Fig. 6.17 Depressor Anguli Oris muscle and the inferior labial artery

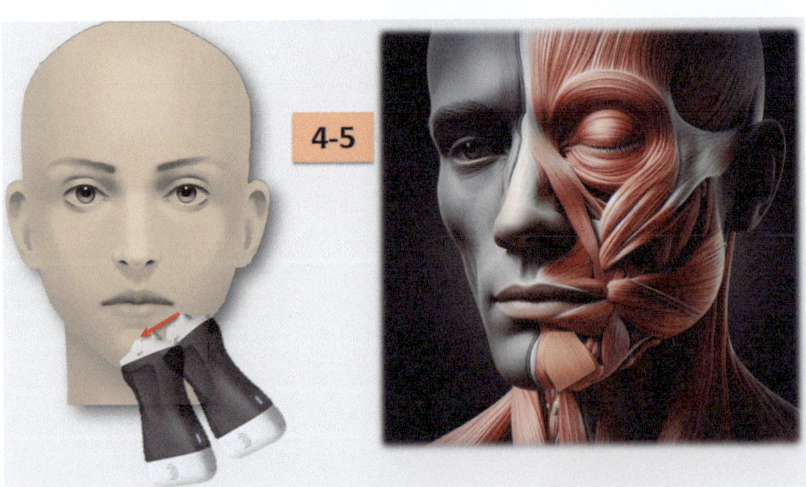

Fig. 6.18 Depressor Labii Inferioris muscle on ultrasound Move from Point 4 the DAO, to the anterior segement of the mid chin, to visualize the DLI muscle, just deep to DAO and the mentalis muscle the most medial muscle in relation to the DAO

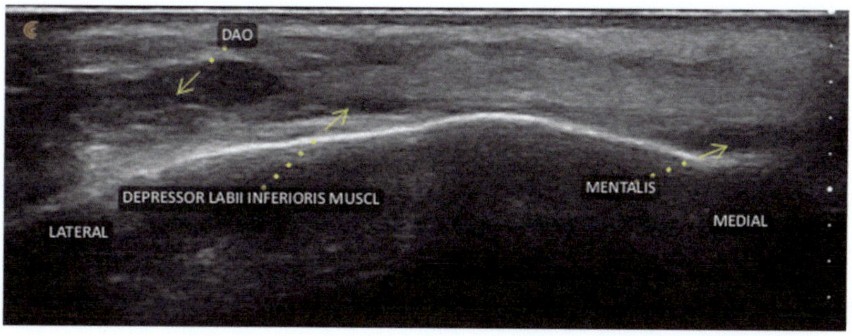

Fig. 6.19 Depressor Labii Inferioris muscle in relation to Depressor Anguli Oris and mentalis muscle

6.1.7 Mentalis Muscle

Transducer in transverse orientation, midpoint of the transducer aligned with the midpoint of the lower chin, approximately 1 cm superior to the mandibular body. The two thin hypoechoic bands seen on either side of the midpoint represent the two bellies of mentalis (Fig. 6.20). **Move from point 5 to point 6**	Fig. 6.20 Transverse view of the mentalis muscle
From the transverse position at DAO, glide transducer to more antero-medial until it is at the midpoint of the chin in the anterior plane. Anatomical variations of the mentalis muscle bellies are found, most common is bilateral bands on either side of the midpoint of the chin (Fig. 6.21). Also consider the curved surface of the pogonion, the transducer should be tilted until it is perpendicular to the muscle belly to prevent anisotropy.	Fig. 6.21 Variants of the mentalis muscle

6.1.8 Superior and Inferior Labial Arteries and the Orbicularis Oris Muscle

Transducer in transverse orientation, place mid midpoint of the transducer at the oral commissure, the facial artery should be located 1.5–2 cm lateral to the oral commissure. At this point it is referred to as the "naked facial artery". Locate the facial artery and trace it from the lateral edge of the lips onto the outer border of the superior vermilion. (Fig. 6.22) Using color Doppler, a tortuous, large pulsating vessel is noted within the subcutaneous layer both within and below the orbicularis oris muscle belly. In the midline, within the philtral columns, columellar arteries may be identified as they branch off superiorly toward the nose from the superior labial artery.	Fig. 6.22 Facial artery branching off to labial arteries
Transverse transducer, with the transducer surface along the vermillion border. The superior labial artery is demonstrated in length (fig. 48). Depending on its course. The depth and entire length may differ amongst patients. Note on image a small columellar artery branch extending from the main superior labial artery (Fig. 6.23).	Fig. 6.23 Superior labial artery on US Fig. 6.24 Inferior labial artery on US
The inferior labial artery is noted near the DAO muscle, lying deep and lateral to the DAO (Fig. 6.24) The artery then traverses towards the lower lip (Fig. 6.25).	Fig. 6.25 Inferior labial artery in relation to DAO

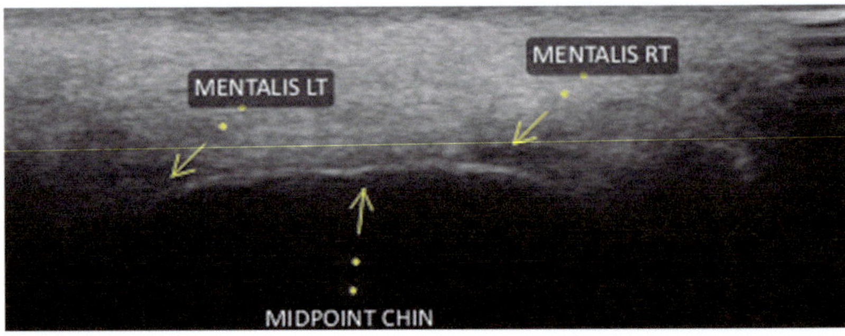

Fig. 6.20 Transverse view of mentalis muscle

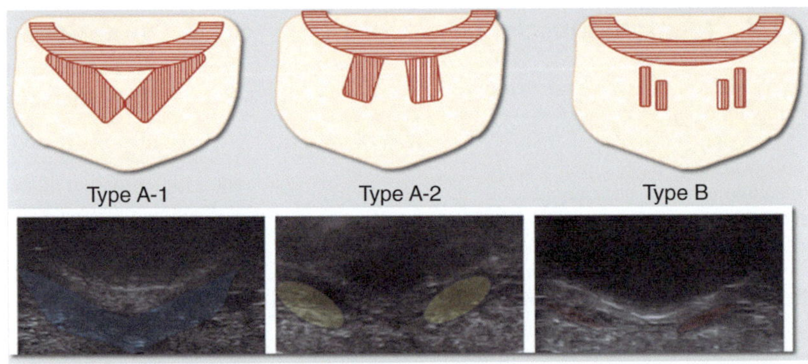

Fig. 6.21 Variants of mentalis muscle

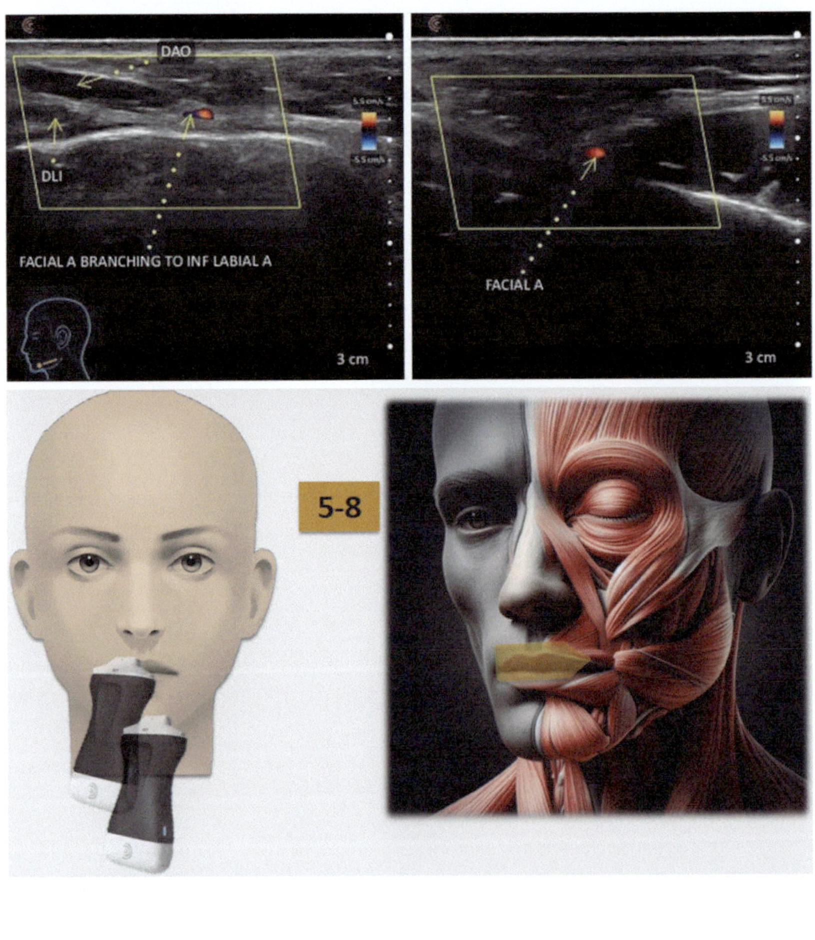

Fig. 6.22 Facial artery branching off to the labial arteries
Move from the mentalis muscle (Point 5) superior along the vermilion border of the lips to visualize the orbicularis oris mucles

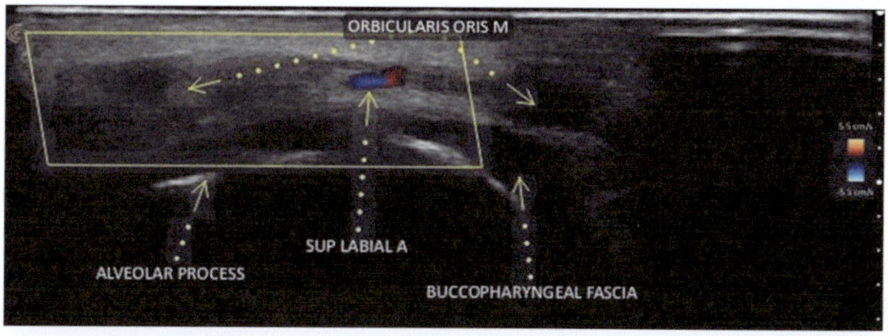

Fig. 6.23 Superior labial artery on ultrasound

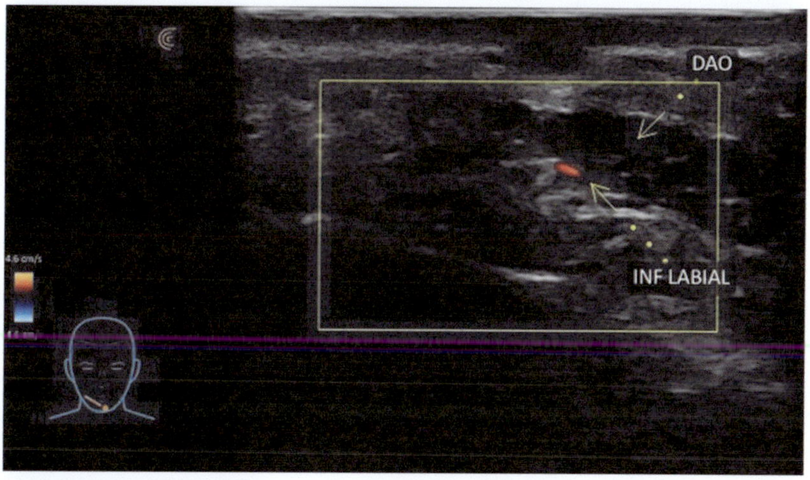

Fig. 6.25 Inferior labial artery in relation to Depressor Anguli Oris muscle
The Inferior labial artery provides a demarcation site between DAO and DLI muscles when Color Doppler is applied

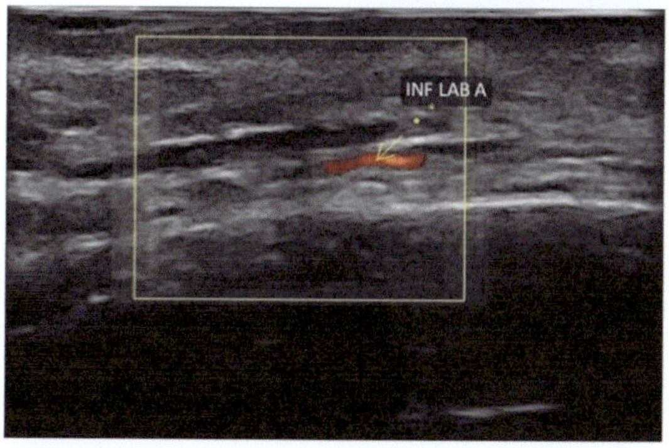

Fig. 6.24 Inferior labial artery on ultrasound
Inferior labial artery is in close proximity to the Depressor labii inferioris muscle (hypoechoic band just superior to artery)

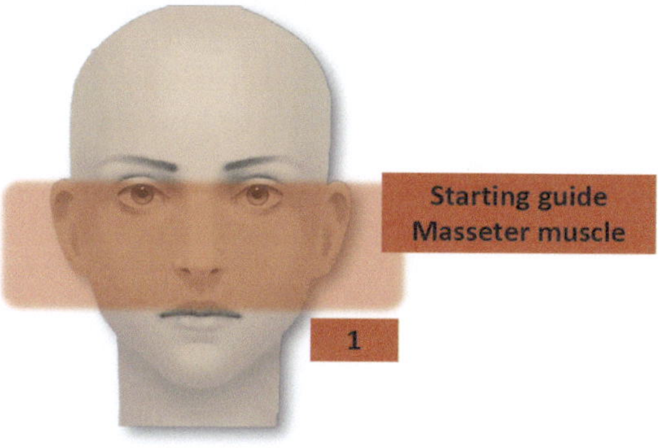

Fig. 6.26 Sonographic stepwise approach to the midface
For the midface, the starting point remains the masseter muscle as point 1, whereafter, the steps move onto the zygomaticus arch

6.2 Midface

Each section of the face is approached using a stepwise approach to sonographic imaging, with easy-to-identify, surface anatomy markers to help discern between key target areas during imaging.

For the midface, the masseter muscle (Fig. 6.26) followed by the zygomatic arch and then medial canthus of the eye and nasolabial fold serves as the starting point for the ultrasound protocol.

6.2.1 Zygomaticus Major Muscle

Tips: *The transducer is placed in transverse orientation along the zygomatic arch. Foot of the transducer resting on the zygomatic arch*	
Place the transducer in the transverse plane on the zygomatic arch, with the midpoint of the transducer aligned with the lateral canthus. The muscle noted on the zygomatic arch is the zygomaticus major muscle (Fig. 6.27).	Fig. 6.27 Zygomaticus major muscle on US
Place the transducer in transverse with its midpoint on the anterior border of the masseter muscle 1 cm superior to the mandible. Glide the transducer from inferior to superior with the foot of the transducer in line with the oral commissure and the heel in the direction of the zygomatic arch. Once at the zygomatic arch rotate the toe of the transducer in a clockwise direction in the direction of the oral commissure until the Zygomaticus major is identified. Zygomaticus major is the first thin hypoechoic band seen at the superior end of the masseter muscle best seen in an oblique plane. (Fig. 6.28)	Fig. 6.28 Zygomaticus major muscle in relation to masseter muscle

6.2.2 Zygomaticus Minor Muscle

The transducer is positioned with its foot along the lateral orbital rim, and the heel is tilted toward the nasolabial fold. The thicker muscle belly, situated beneath the orbicularis oculi muscle, corresponds to the zygomaticus minor muscle. (Fig. 6.29)	Fig. 6.29 Zygomaticus minor muscle in relation to orbicularis oculi muscle
By maintaining the transducer's foot on the lateral orbital rim, the heel of the transducer is directed toward the oral commissure. It is important to note that the muscle overlying the zygomatic bone is, indeed, the zygomaticus minor muscle (Fig. 6.30)	Fig. 6.30 Zygomaticus minor muscle in relation to the zygoma

6.2.3 Angular Artery and Vein

The transducer foot is set on the medial canthus and aligned along the nasolabial fold, just lateral to the nasalis muscle. Colour Doppler is selected, the colour box is angled to 60°. Adjust colour gain and scale (approximately cm/sec) to ensure the small arterial flow rates are visualized clearly. The angular artery lies in close relation to Levator Labii Superioris Alaeque Nasalis (LLSAN) muscle (Fig. 6.31) With the foot of the transducer remaining on the medial can thus, swivel the transducer heel in small increments more laterally to visualize the angular vein. Light pressure is essential so as not to compress the angular vein. The angular vein lies in the nasojugal fold (need a reference here). To confirm if the angular vein is visualized, spectral imaging can be used to showcase a venous waveform. ***Angular artery is medial to the angular vein and seen more lateral***	Fig. 6.31 Angular artery in relation to LLSAN
The angular artery (Fig. 6.32) When color gain is increased, the lateral nasal branches are also visualized.	Fig. 6.32 Angular artery through use of Color Doppler

6.2.4 Levator Labii Superioris Alaeque Nasalis (LLSAN) in Relation to Angular Artery

Tips: *The transducer foot rests on the medial canthus of the eye and the heel of the transducer lies along the nasojugal fold.* *The transducer is tilted slightly medial to see the nasal cartilage in profile with LLSAN lying just above the infraorbital fat pad.* *Overactivation of the LLSAN in conjunction with the orbicularis oculi produces the so-called bunny/wolf lines. These lines are found clinically in a diagonal direction at right angles to the contraction of th LLSAN and orbicularis oculi.*	
Position 1: From medial canthus to nasojugal fold (Fig. 6.33)	Fig. 6.33 LLSAN visualized in Position 1
Position 2: From medial canthus turning transducer heel to lateral and transverse orientation, from lateral to medial the muscle bellies noted are levator anguli oris muscle, levator labii superioris muscle and most medial is LLSAN (Fig. 6.34).	Fig. 6.34 LLSAN visualized in Position 2

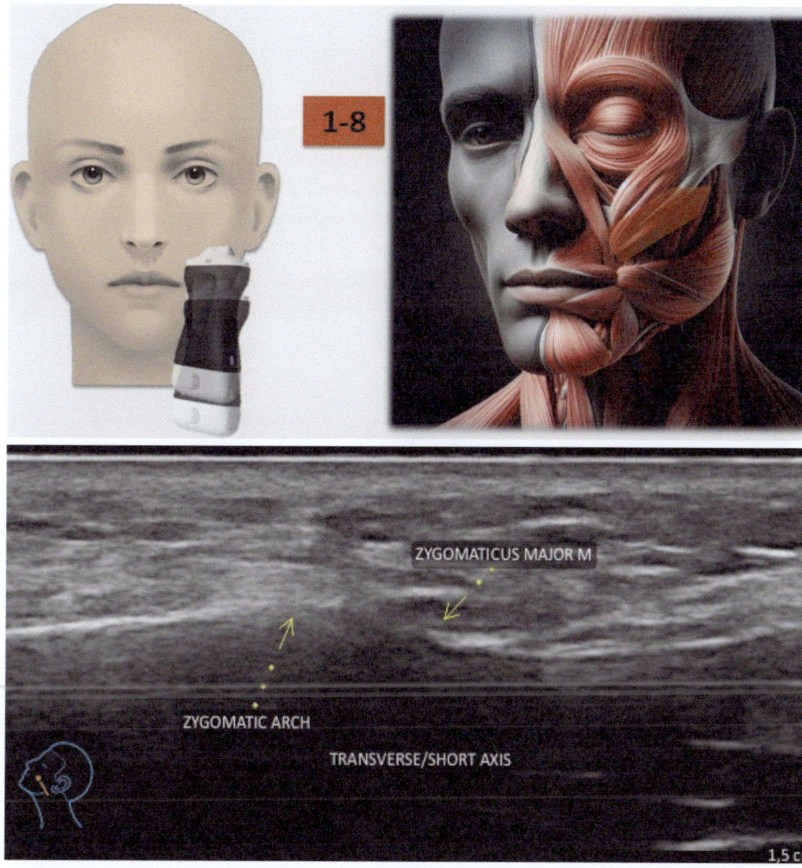

Fig. 6.27 Zygomaticus major muscle on ultrasound
Move from point 1 to 8 to visualize the zygomaticus arch. This is through upwards superior gliding of the probe towards the cheek's bony margin

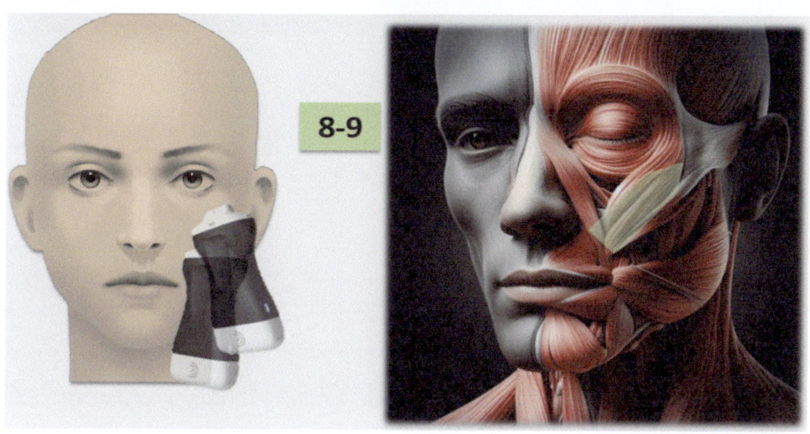

Fig. 6.28 Zygomaticus major muscle in relation to masseter muscle
Move from the zygomatic arch (point 8) with a heel toe motion. The heel (medial part of the probe) remains seated on the zygomatic arch and the toe (lateral part of probe) is swivelled superior to visualize the zygomaticus major muscle in profile

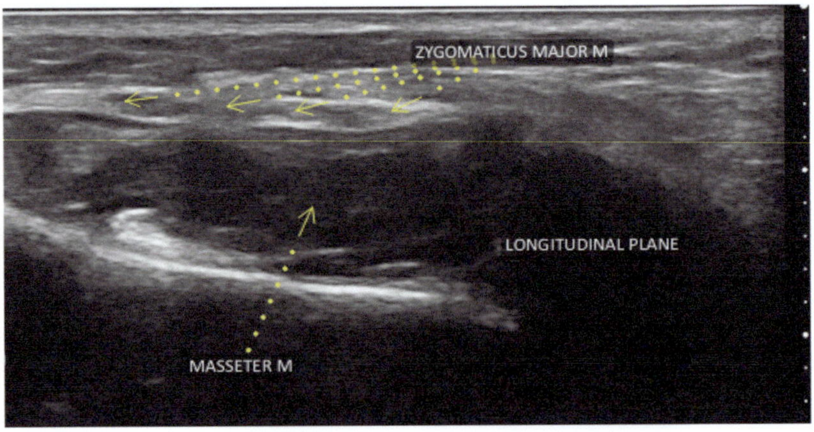

Fig. 6.29 Zygomaticus minor muscle in relation to orbicularis oculis muscle

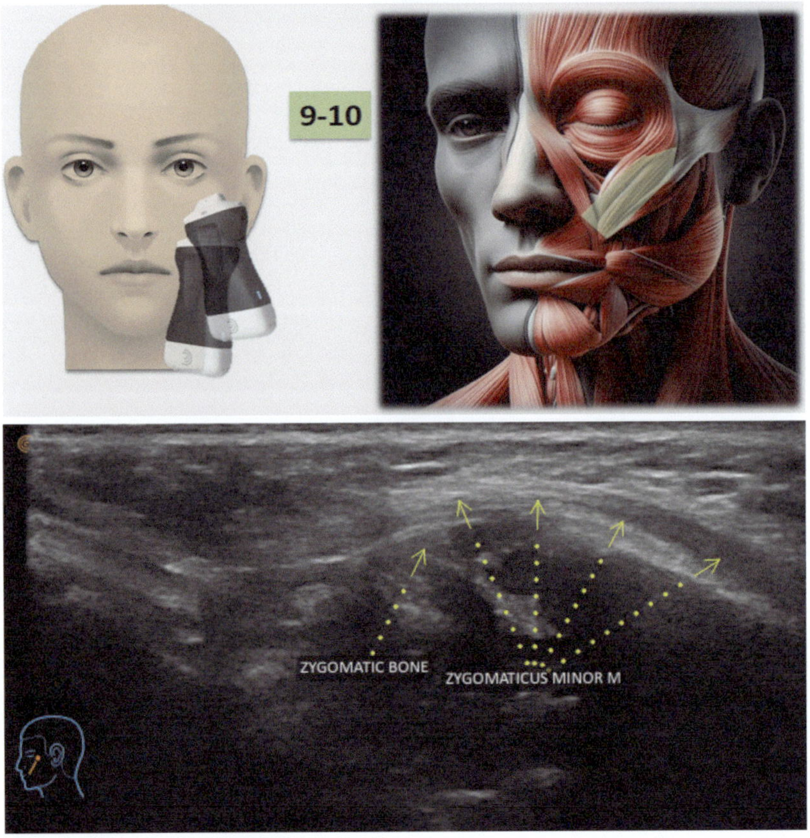

Fig. 6.30 Zygomaticus minor muscle in relation to the zygoma
Move from point 9 (zygomaticus major muscle) to point 10 with the toe of the probe angled towards the lateral canthus of the eye
Orbicularis oculi in relation to zygomaticus muscles
Move probe from point 10 to point 11, by placing the probe onto the inferior orbital rim in a transverse orientation

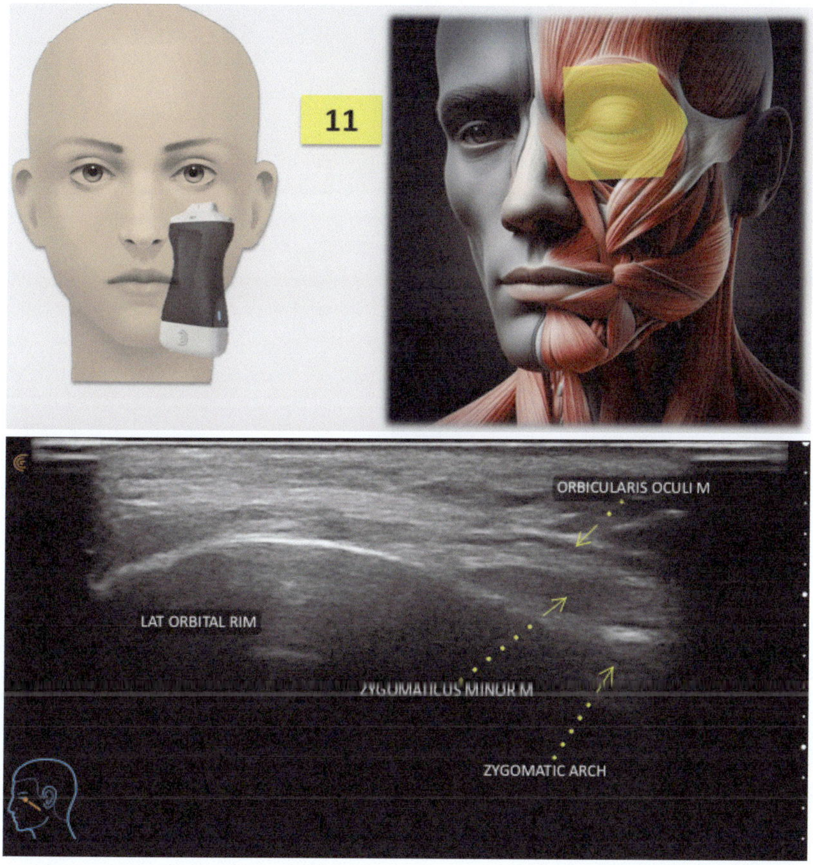

Fig. 6.30 (continued)

Fig. 6.31 Angular artery in relation to levator labii superioris alaeque nasalis
Point A is the imaginary line drawn from the medial canthus of the eye towards to nasiolabial fold, this is the starting point to visualise all the muscles in relation to the angular artery and vein

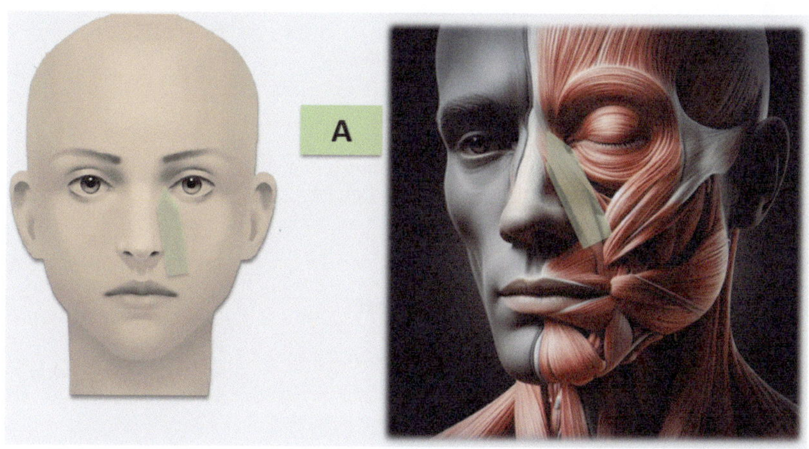

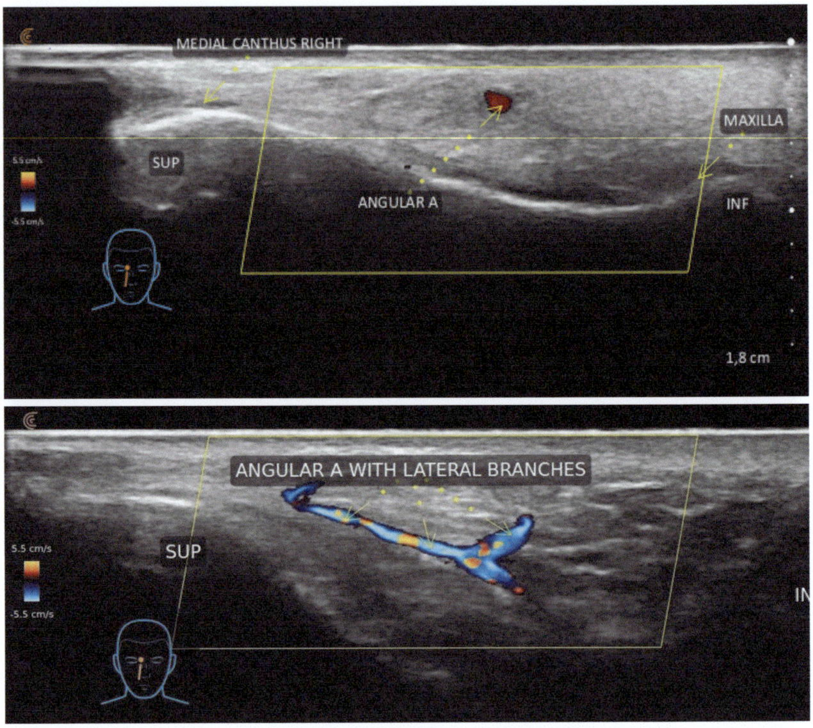

Fig. 6.32 Angular artery through use of Color Doppler

6.2.5 Nasalis Muscle

Tips:

The transducer is placed in a longitudinal plane at an oblique coronal plane along the nasal cartilage. Nasalis arises from the maxilla and inserts onto the nasal bone.

Contraction of transverse portion of nasalis compresses the nasal aperture, whereas the dilator naris muscle enlarges the nostril.

Transducer in an oblique coronal plane, the transducer can be glided from LLSAN and moved more medially and tilted along the nasal cartilage. (Fig. 6.35)	Fig. 6.35 Nasalis muscle in oblique coronal plane

6.2.6 Temporal Fossa and the Ten Layers Visualized on Ultrasound

Tips:

The transducer is placed along the zygomatic arch in the transverse plane and moved more cranially, with the temporalis muscle noted within the temporal fossa.

Transducer foot is placed at the K-point and the heel is in the longitudinal plane to visualize temporalis muscle in its long axis, the most distal portion is noted beneath the zygomatic arch and the upper masseter muscle. (Fig. 6.36) The 10 layers are from superficial to deep: 1. Skin 2. Subcutaneous fat 3. Superficial temporal fascia 4. Loose alveolar tissue 5. Superficial lamina of the deep temporal fascia 6. Superficial temporal fat 7. Deep lamina of the deep temporal fascia 8. Temporal extension of the Bichat fat 9. Temporalis muscle 10. Temporal bone	Fig. 6.36 The ten layers from superficial to deep

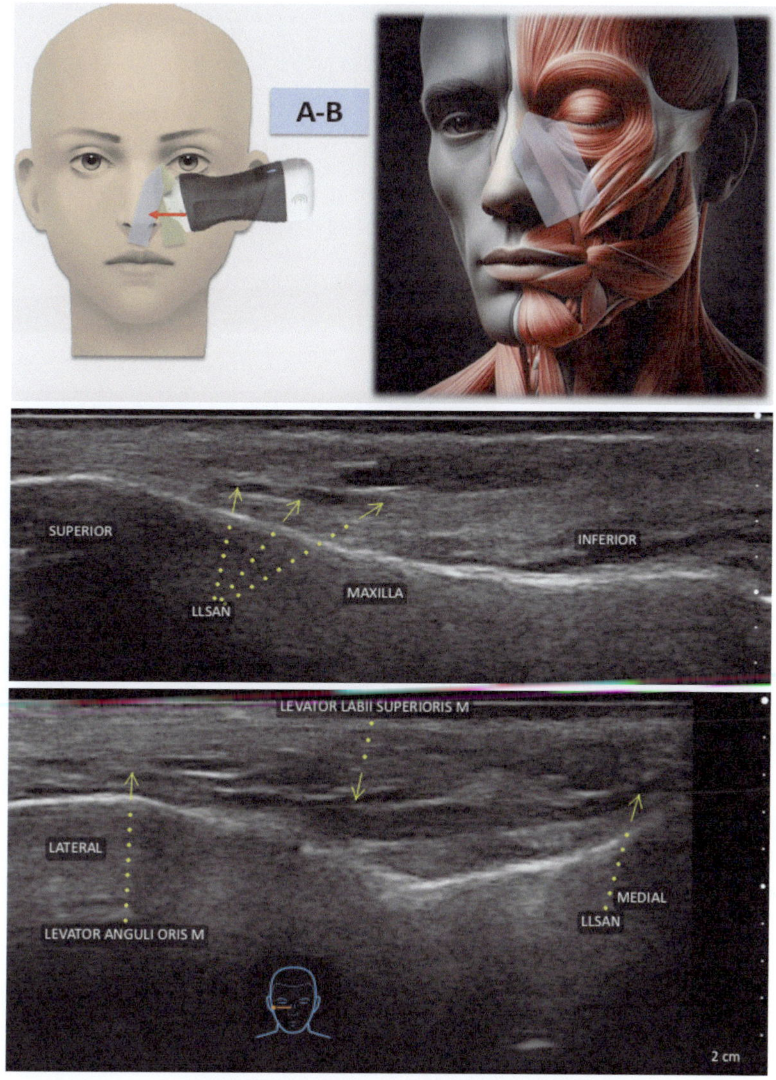

Fig. 6.33 Levator labii superioris alaeque nasalis visualized in position 1
Using a heel toe approach, the heel of the probe (most superior part) remains on the medial canthus of the eye, whilst the toe of the probe (most inferior part) swivels towards the far medial aspect of the lateral surface of the nose

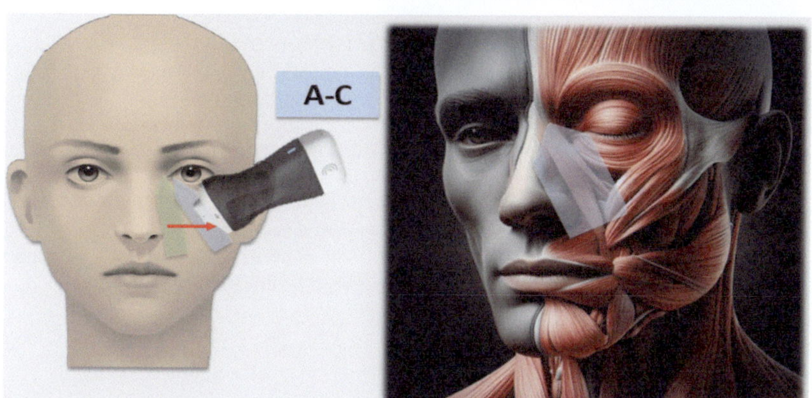

Fig. 6.34 Levator labii superioris alaeque nasalis visualized in position 2
Through use of the heel toe method, the heel of the probe (most superior part) remains on the medial canthus of the eye, and the toe (most inferior part) swivels towards the far lateral aspect of the midface. This motion is done in small increments from Point A to Point C whilst enabling color Doppler to visualise the angular artery and vein

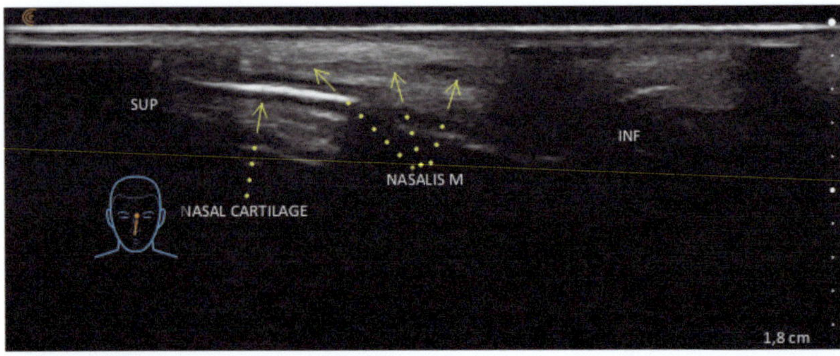

Fig. 6.35 Nasalis muscle in oblique coronal plane

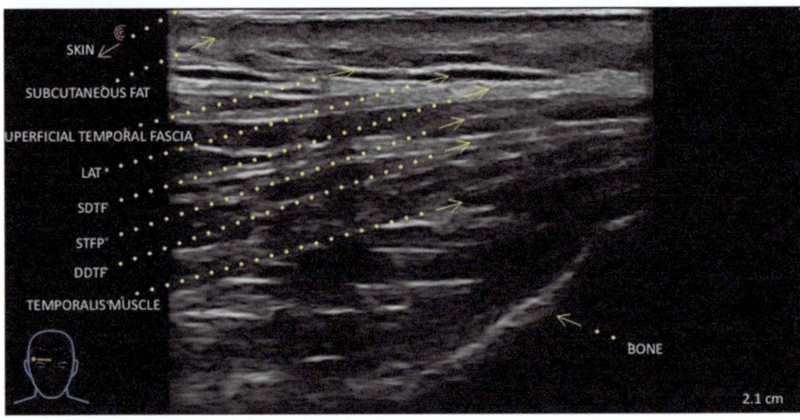

Fig. 6.36 The ten layers from superficial to deep

6.2.7 Temporal Fossa and Associated Vasculature

Tips:

The temporal vessels are easily compressed during sonographic imaging, causing difficulty to visualize. A light touch of the ultrasound surface with a gel standoff pad is required for optimal visualization. The use of increased color gain, and optimal color box steering of 60 degrees is ideal method to use to visualize the vasculature in this region.
Between layers 2–4: Superficial temporal artery
Between layers 5–7 is the middle temporal vein
Between layers 9–10 are the anterior and posterior branches of the deep temporal artery.

Transducer is placed with the foot at the K-point (Fig. 6.37). Colour Doppler is turned on. The heel of the transducer is swiveled from an 11 o'clock position to a 6 o'clock position until the superficial temporal artery is identified in layers 2–3.	Fig. 6.37 K-point in relation to superficial temporal artery
Light pressure should be applied so as not to compress the superficial temporal artery. Power Doppler is ideal to assist in locating the superficial temporal artery (Fig. 6.38) if the STA is not identified on colour Doppler.	Fig. 6.38 Superficial temporal artery
To identify the anterior and posterior branches of the deep temporal artery, place the transducer in transverse on the zygomatic arch. Increase depth on B-mode to be able to see the temporal bone. Place colour Doppler on. (Fig. 6.39)	Fig. 6.39 Anterior and posterior branches of deep temporal artery
Slide the transducer from inferior to superior. Located between layers 9–10, are the anterior branch of the deep temporal artery (Fig. 6.40) Near the superficial temporal artery, is the temporal branch of the facial nerve, noted in cross section as an oval shaped ring with salt and pepper center (Fig. 6.41). Middle temporal vein noted between layers 5–6 (Fig. 6.42).	Fig. 6.40 Anterior branch of deep temporal artery Fig. 6.41 Temporal branch of facial nerve in relation to superficial temporal artery Fig. 6.42 Middle temporal vein

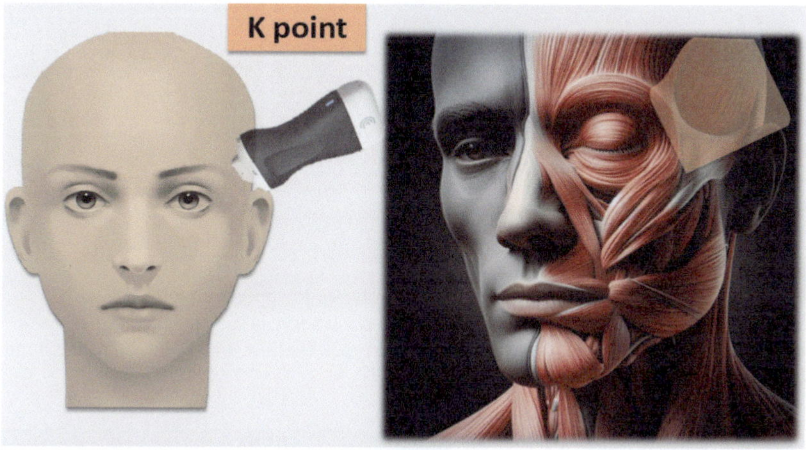

Fig. 6.37 K-point in relation to superficial temporal artery
The so called K point is: Using the K point as a starting guide, the probe is swivelled in small increments from superior to inferior with the heel of the probe (most medial part) remains fixed on the lateral edge of the brow/ lateral orbital rim

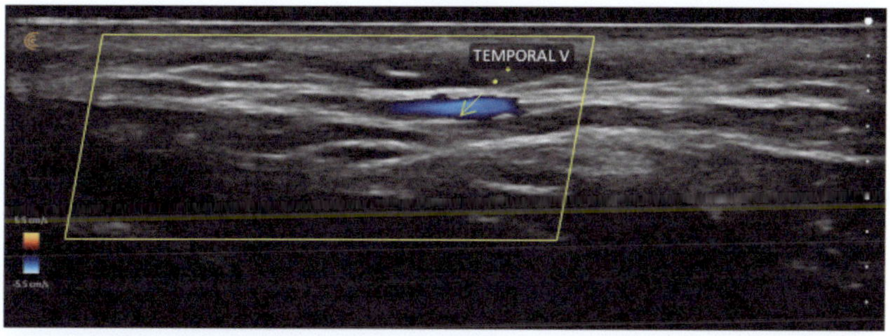

Fig. 6.38 Superficial temporal artery

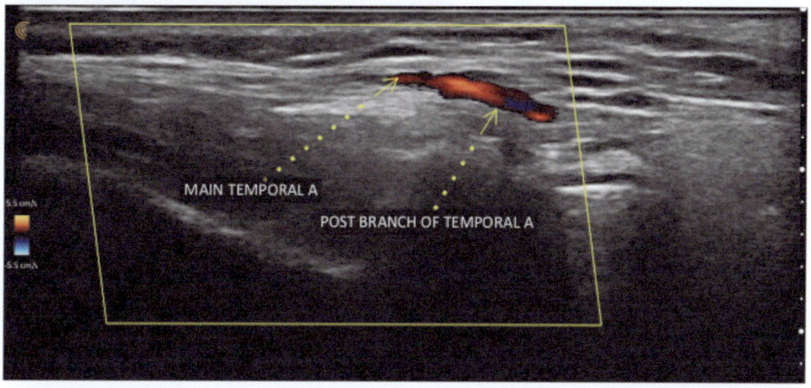

Fig. 6.39 Anterior and posterior branches of the deep temporal artery

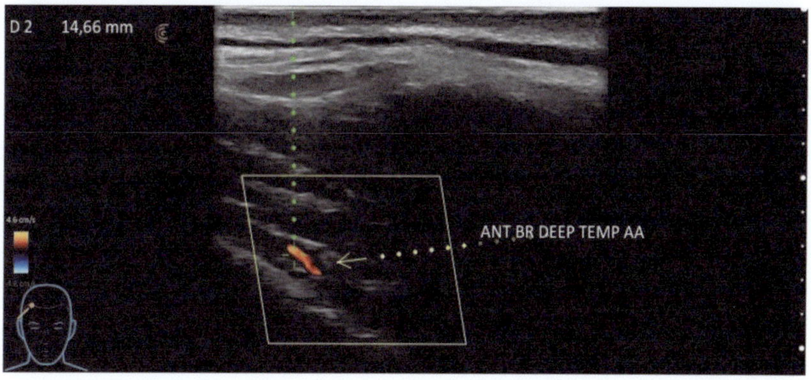

Fig. 6.40 Anterior branch of the deep temporal artery

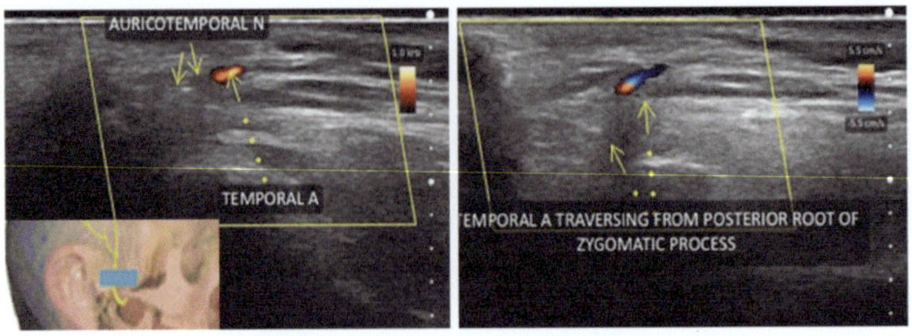

Fig. 6.41 Temporal branch of facial nerve in relation to superficial temporal artery
The salt and pepper appearance of the auricotemporal nerve is seen posterior to the temporal artery using Power Doppler on the left hand image. Small white and black specks (yellow arrow) indicates the neurofascicular pattern of the nerve bundle when visualised in transverse plane

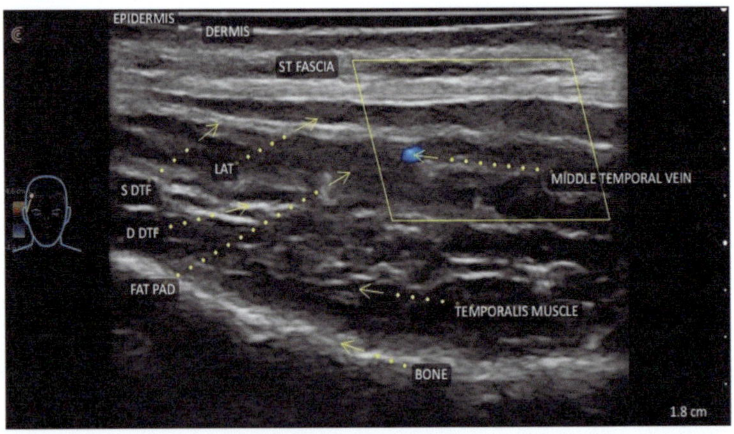

Fig. 6.42 Middle temporal vein

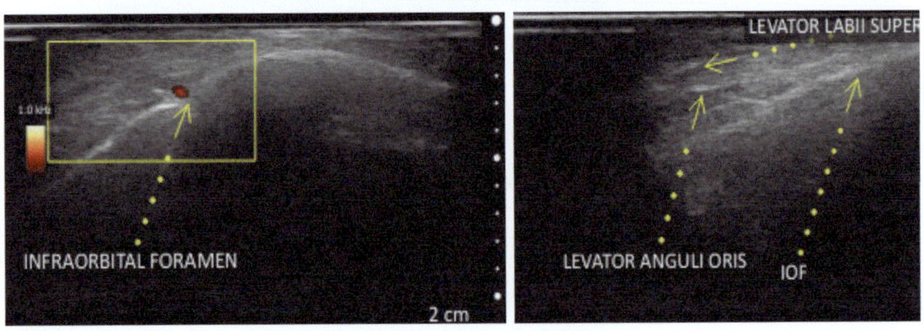

Fig. 6.43 Inferior orbital foramen in transverse plane

6.2.8 Inferior Orbital Foramen

Along the inferior orbital rim, the transducer is placed in transverse orientation with it's midpoint at the midpoint of the eye (pupil). Colour or power Doppler is selected. A small cortical break in the maxilla is noted (Fig. 6.43), where an arterial vessel is noted traversing longitudinal into the cortical break, known as the infraorbital foramen. The two muscles above this level are the levator anguli oris and levator labii superioris muscles	Fig. 6.43 Inferior orbital foramen in transverse plane

6.3 Upper Face

Figure: Stepwise Approach Figure Upper Face

Each section of the face is approached using a stepwise approach to sonographic imaging, with easy-to-identify, surface anatomy markers to help discern between key target areas during imaging.

For the upper face, the glabella (Fig. 6.44) serves as the reference point during imaging.

6.3.1 Frontalis Muscle

Tips: *Aging is associated with horizontal rhytids of the forehead.* *Neurotoxins are commonly used, in the correct patient, to relax the frontalis muscle.* *The frontalis is the sole elevator muscle of the upper face and needs to be injected with caution with neurotoxins to avoid a feeling of heaviness of the brow and a brow drop.*	
The transducer is placed in the transverse plane one finger width cranial to the eyebrow. Frontalis muscle is visible just below the SMAS and above the frontal bone (Fig. 6.45)	Fig. 6.45 Frontalis muscle in transverse plane

6.3.2 Procerus Muscle

Tips: *Patients with supranuclear palsy may present focal dystonia of the procerus muscle, known as the procerus sign.* *Neurotoxin injection of the procerus muscle is used to reduce horizontal furrow lines at the bridge of the nose.*	
Transducer is placed in transverse on the nasion, just proximal to the nasalis muscle. Procerus is noted over the frontal bone and deep to the SMAS (Fig. 6.46).	Fig. 6.46 Procerus muscle in transverse plane

6.3.3 Corrugator Supercilli Muscle

Tips: *This is known as the frowning muscle.* *Responsible for vertical rhytids or so-called "11's" on the forehead.* *The use of neuromodulator in the corrugator supercilii muscle is a common aesthetic treatment target.*	
The transducer is placed at a 45-degree angle along the edge of the medial eyebrow and can be assessed dynamically through active frowning of the upper face to validate presence of the corrugator muscle. The corrugator is noted deep to the depressor supercilii muscle with its lateral border deep to the orbicularis oculi muscle (Fig. 6.47). An anatomical landmark is the supraorbital foramen noted deep to the corrugator muscle, along the cortical ridge. Note the branch of the supraorbital artery near the corrugator muscle along its medial border (Fig. 6.48).	Fig. 6.47 Corrugator supercilii muscle in relation to depressor supercilii muscle Fig. 6.48 Corrugator supercilii muscle in relation to the supraorbital artery

6.3.4 Orbicularis Oculi Muscle

Tips: *The orbicularis oculi muscle plays an important role in the blink reflex, evaluating the integrity of the trigeminal and facial nerves.* *The muscle is commonly targeted with neurotoxin for the treatment of lateral canthal lines or crow's feet.*	
Transducer placed either along the superior or inferior orbital rim in a transverse plane. The thin hypoechoic band noted just below the thin layer of subcutaneous soft tissue is the orbicularis oculi muscle (Fig. 6.49). The SubOrbicularis oculi fat (SOOF) is noted deep to the orbicularis oculi muscle in the infra orbital area.	Fig. 6.49 Orbicularis oculi muscle in the transverse plane

6.3.5 Superior Orbital Foramen and Supratrochlear Notch/Foramen

For the supraorbital foramen: Place transducer in transverse orientation (Fig. 6.50), with the midpoint aligned to the midpoint of the eyebrow/superior orbital rim. Glide the transducer below the eyebrow ridge and tilt slightly upwards until a cortical break is noted on the orbital rim. Place power doppler over the area, and increase the color gain, to visualize the supraorbital artery traversing through the foramen.	Fig. 6.50 Supra-orbital foramen in transverse plane

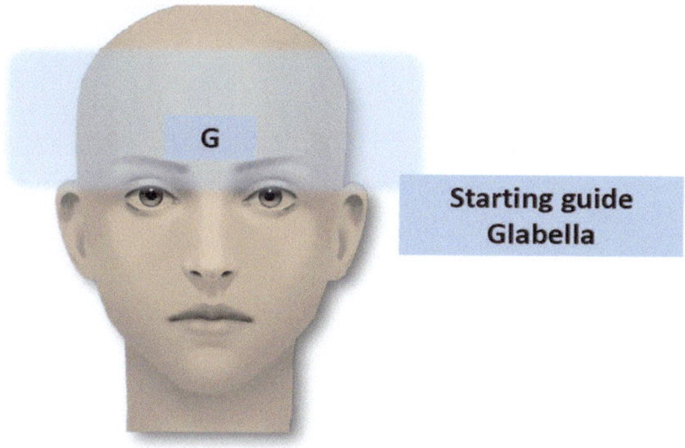

Fig. 6.44 Sonographic stepwise approach to the upper face
The starting point for the upper face is the glabella, probe is placed in transverse or saggital orientation on top of the glabella surface (G)

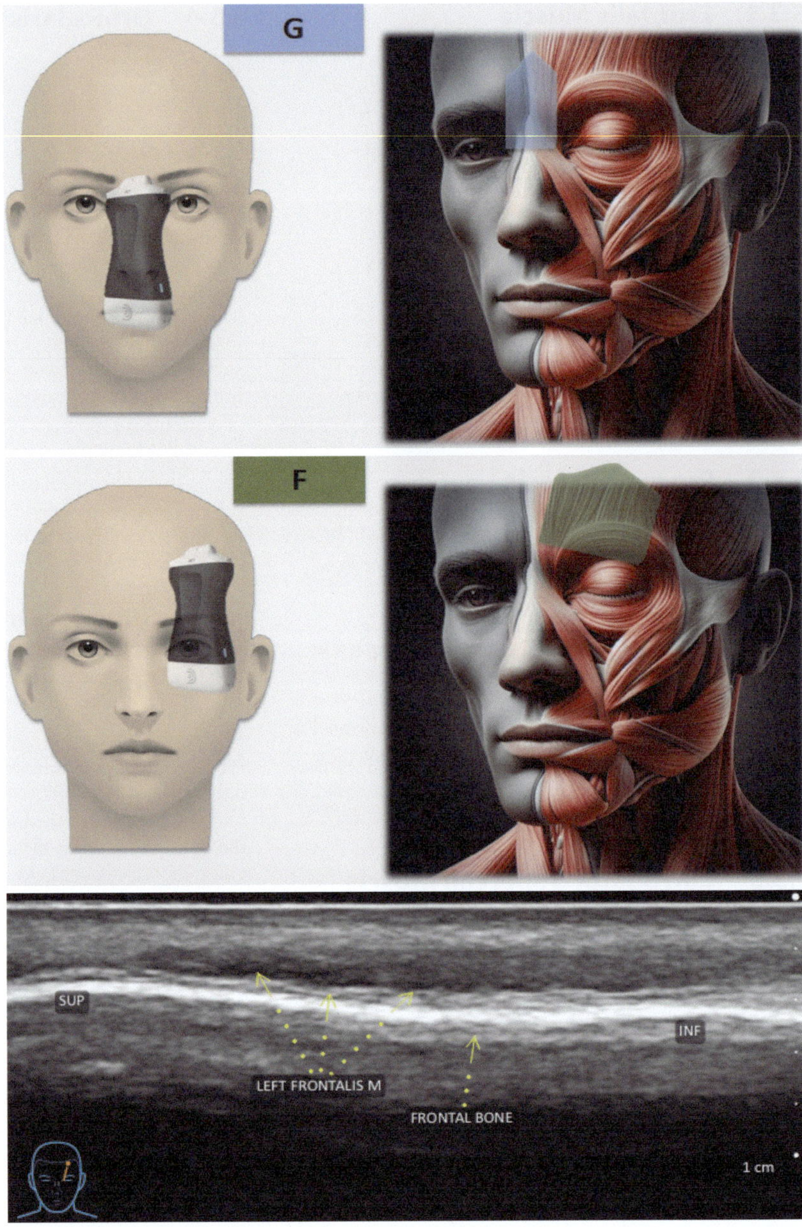

Fig. 6.45 Frontalis muscle in transverse plane
Image 1: Moving from the glabella, the probe is glided superior and lateral towards the metopian line to visualize the frontalis muscle
Image 2: Probe is glided lateral and superior to visualize the frontalis muscle
Image 3: Sonongraphic representation of the frontalis muscle in transverse plane

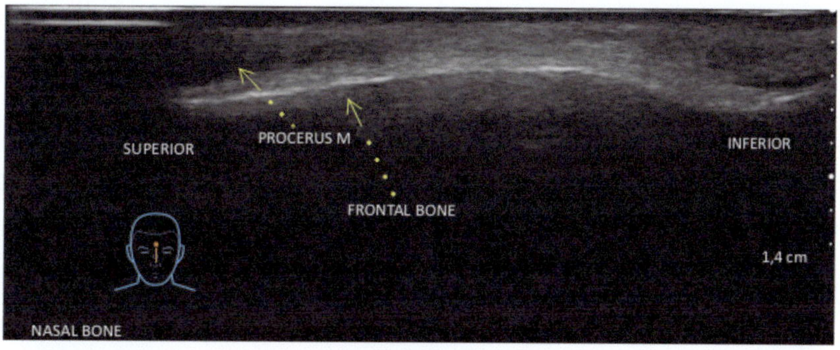

Fig. 6.46 Procerus muscle in transverse plane

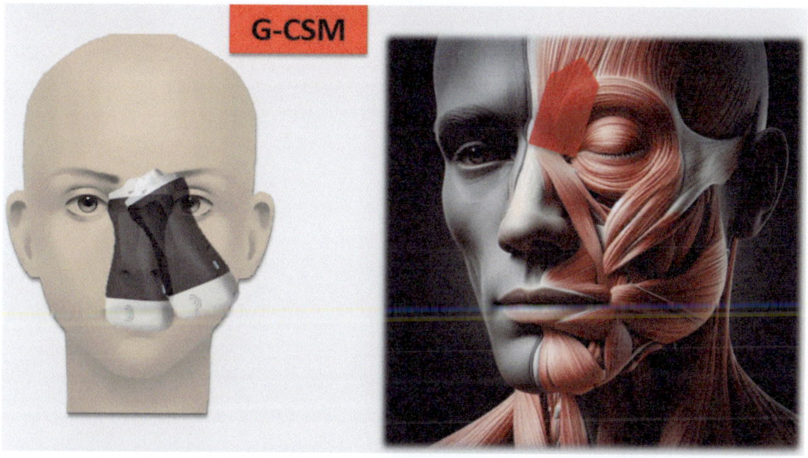

Fig. 6.47 Corrugator supercilli muscle in relation to depressor supercilli muscle Moving the probe from point G to CSM requires a slight angle of the probe along the medial orbital rim, so that the probe runs in the same anatomical plane as the corrugator supercilli muscle (CSM)

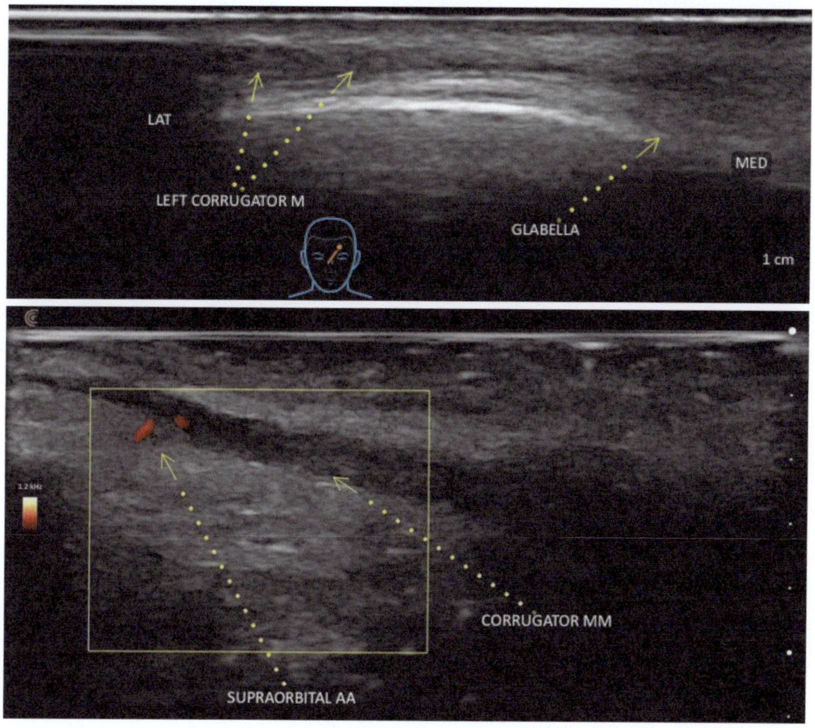

Fig. 6.48 Corrugator supercilli muscle in relation to the supra orbital artery

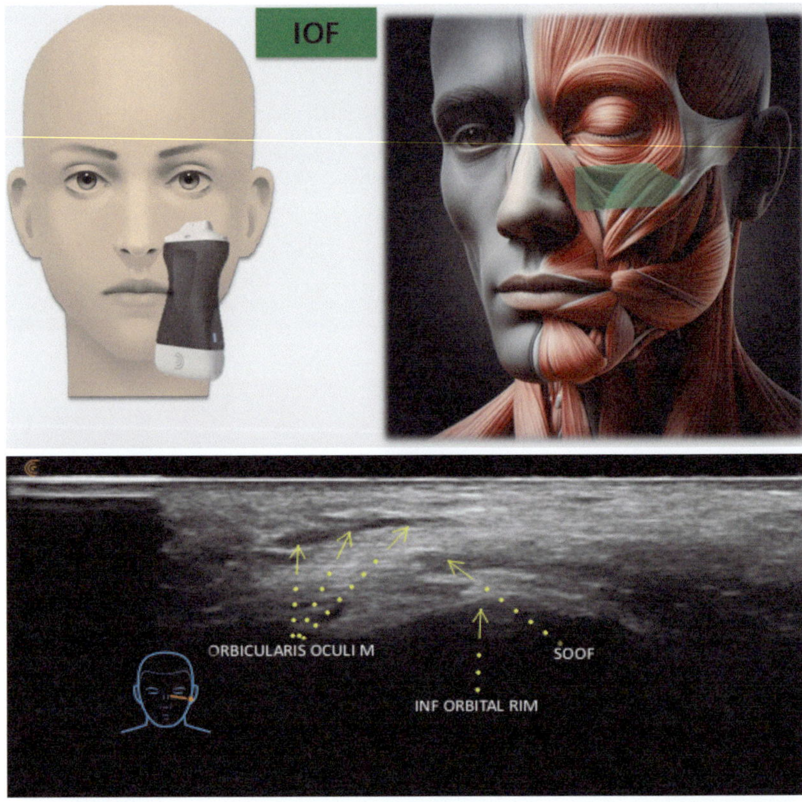

Fig. 6.49 Orbicularis oculi muscle in the transverse plane
Placing the probe in line with the midpupillary line and on top of the infraorbital rim, Power doppler is applied to ensure the infraorbital artery traversing the foramen is visualized

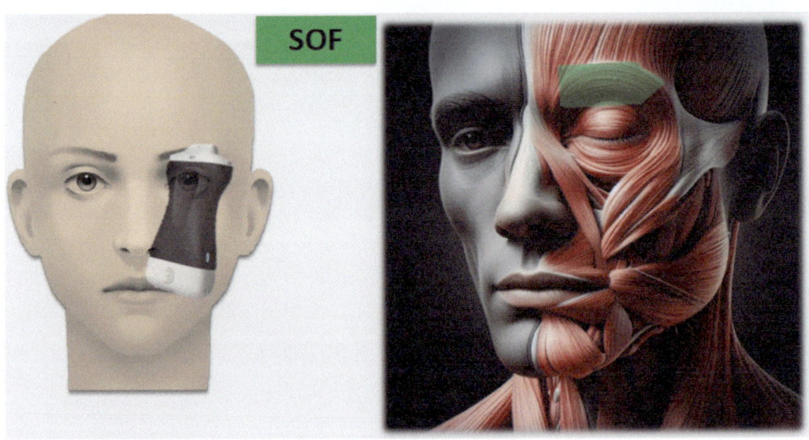

Fig. 6.50 Supra orbital foramen in transverse plane
Placing the probe in line with the midpupillary line and on top of the supraorbital rim, Power doppler is applied to ensure the supraorbital artery traversing the foramen is visualized

Supratrochlear notch: Place the transducer in an oblique longitudinal plane (Fig. 6.51), in the deep superior medial ridge of the orbital rim. Slightly angle the transducer towards the glabellar region until a cortical break is noted along the medial orbital surface. (Fig. 6.52) Place power doppler over the area, and increase the color gain, to visualize the supratrochlear artery traversing through the foramen. In this image the supratrochlear nerve is also noted as a salt and pepper appearance just lateral to the artery. The cranial portion of the corrugator supercilii muscle is also noted in profile (Fig. 6.53).	Fig. 6.51 Superficial temporal nerve in oblique longitudinal plane Fig. 6.52 The use of power Doppler in visualizing the foramen Fig. 6.53 Supratrochlear nerve in relation to the superficial temporal nerve

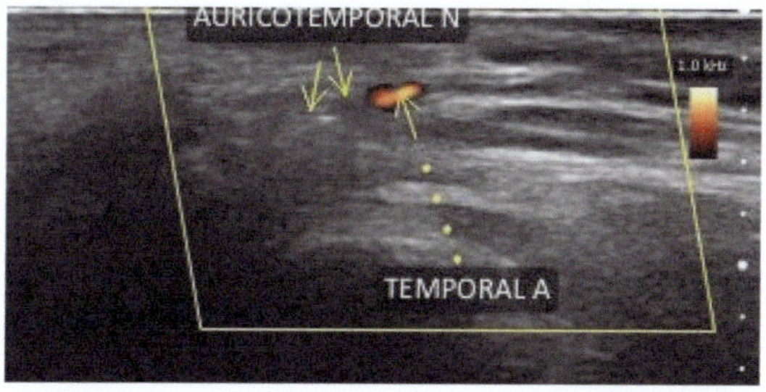

Fig. 6.51 Superficial temporal nerve in oblique longitudinal plane

Fig. 6.52 The use of power Doppler in visualizing the foramen

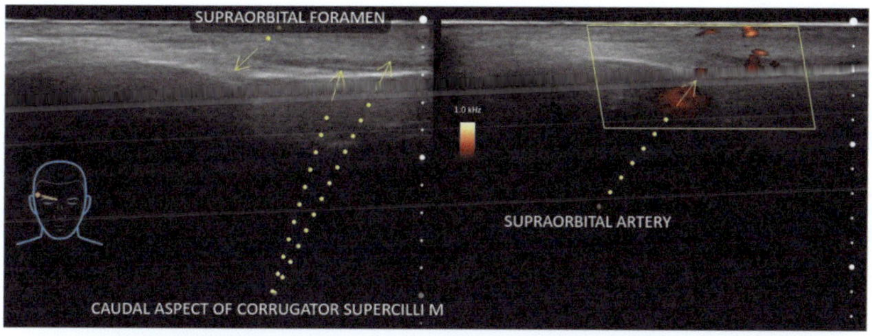

Fig. 6.53 Supratrochlear nerve in relation to the superficial temporal nerve

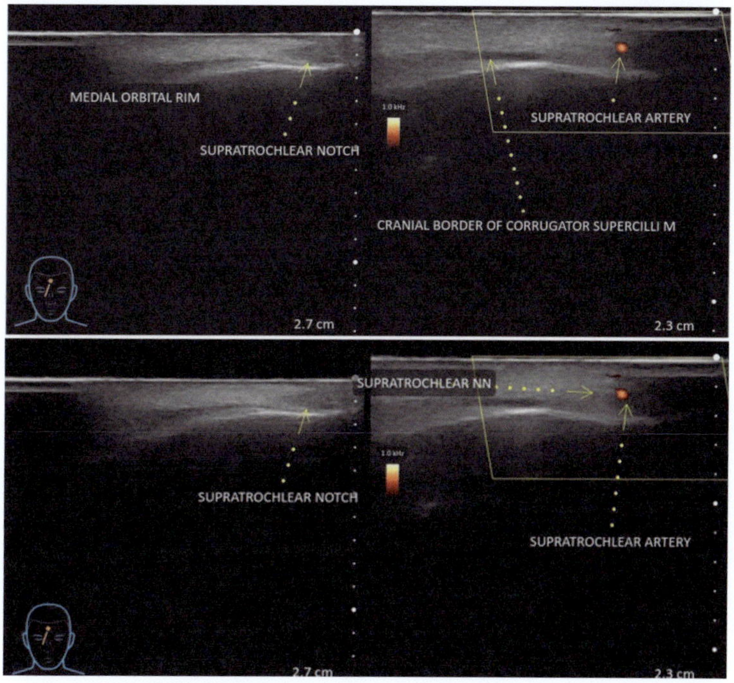

Appendix

Pocketbook Atlas for Facial Aesthetics

Lower Face (Fig. A.1)

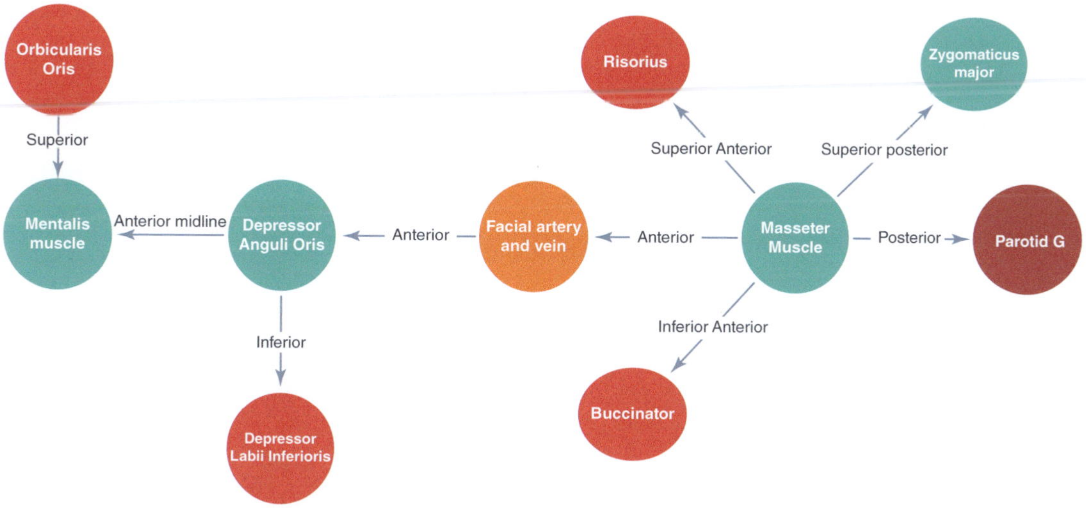

Fig. A.1 Flowchart of the lower face

K. Malherbe, S. Roberts, *Ultrasound Protocol for Facial Aesthetics*,
https://doi.org/10.1007/978-3-031-75949-9

Upper Face (Fig. A.2)

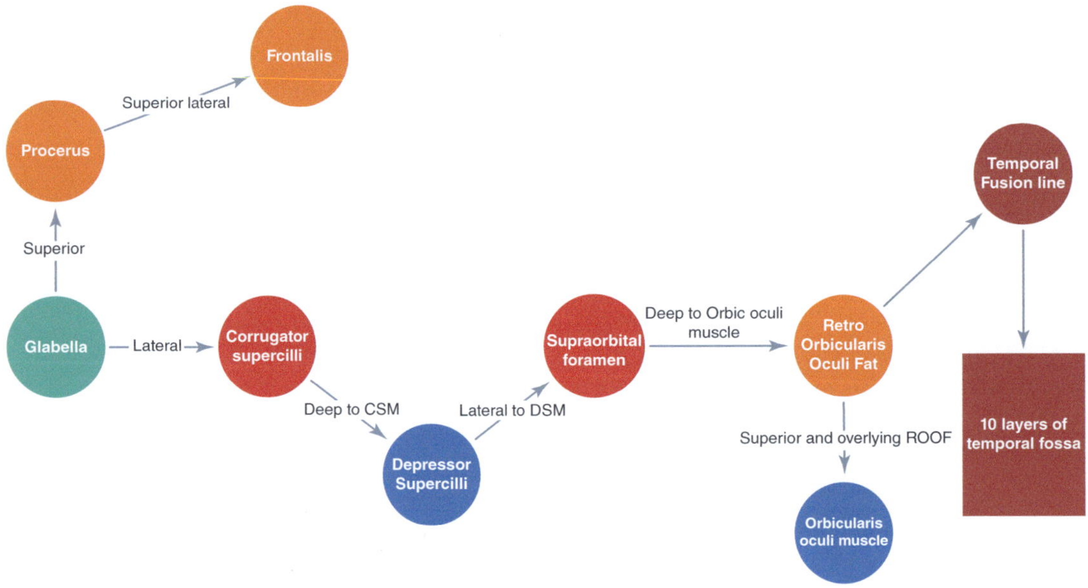

Fig. A.2 Flowchart of the upper face

Midface (Fig. A.3)

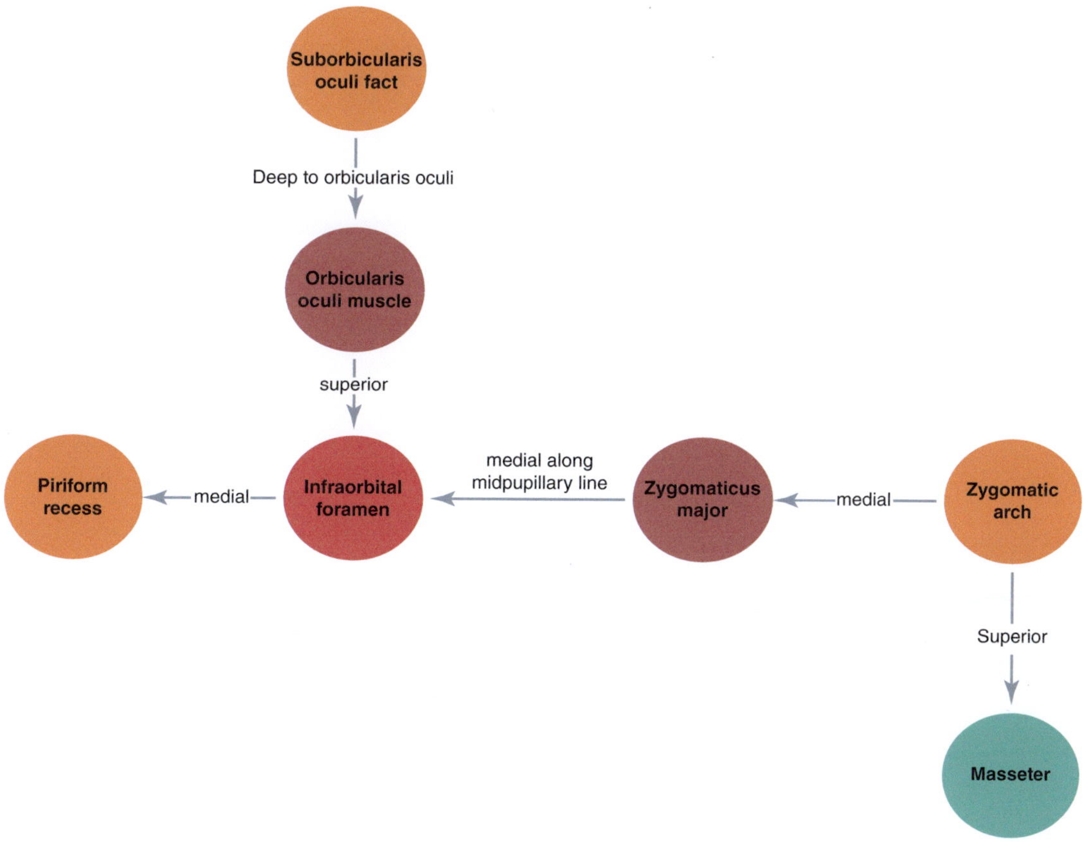

Fig. A.3 Flowchart of the midface

Facial Artery Course (Fig. A.4)

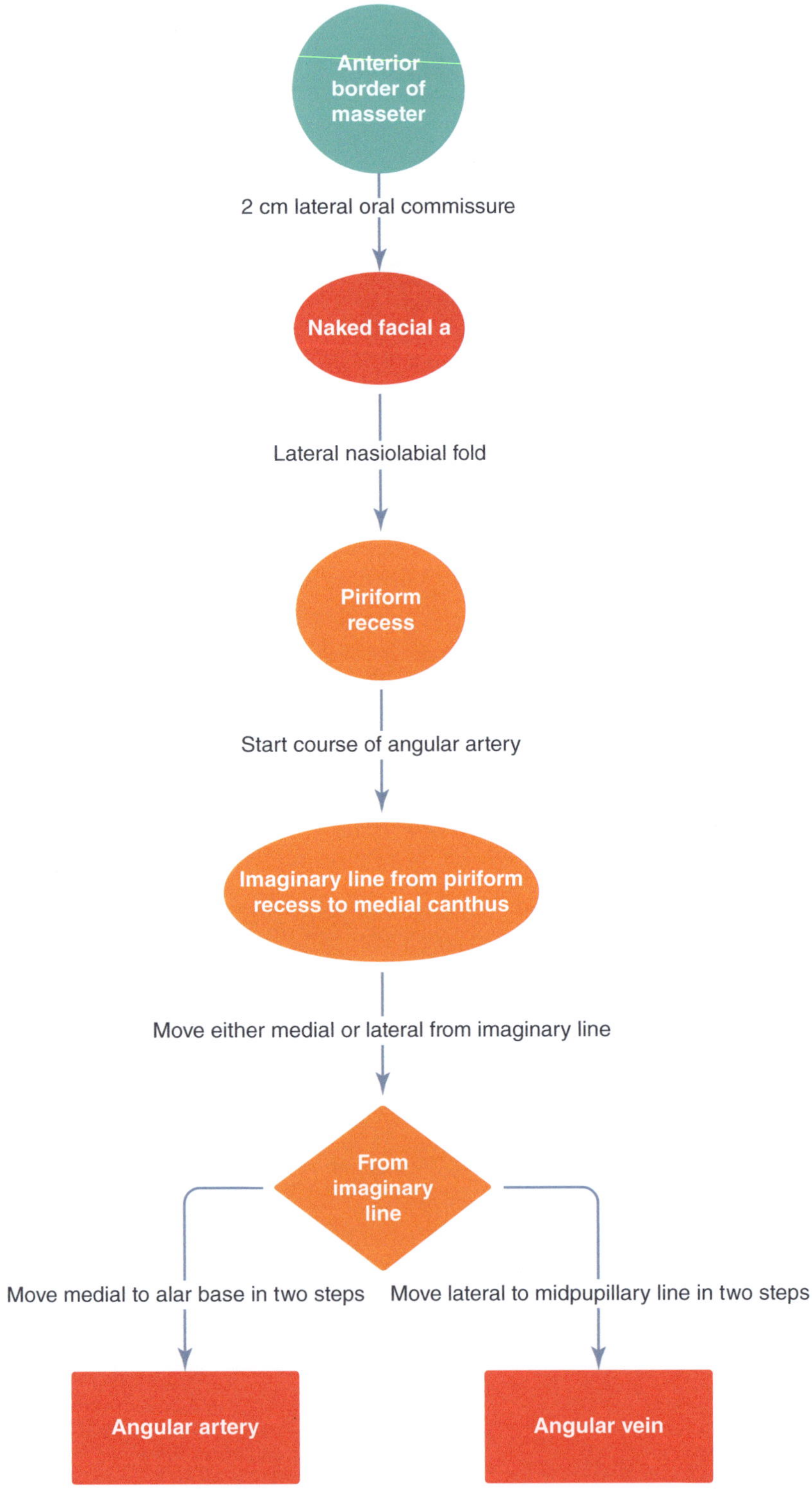

Fig. A.4 Facial artery course flow chart

External Carotid Artery and its Branches (Fig. A.5)

Some **A**natomists **L**ove **F**reaking **O**ut **P**oor **M**edical **S**tudents

SALFOPMS

S: superior thyroid artery (first branch proximal to common carotid artery)
A: ascending pharyngeal artery
L: lingual artery
F: facial artery
O: occipital artery
P: posterior auricular artery
M: maxillary artery (largest terminal branch)
S: superficial temporal artery (terminal branch)

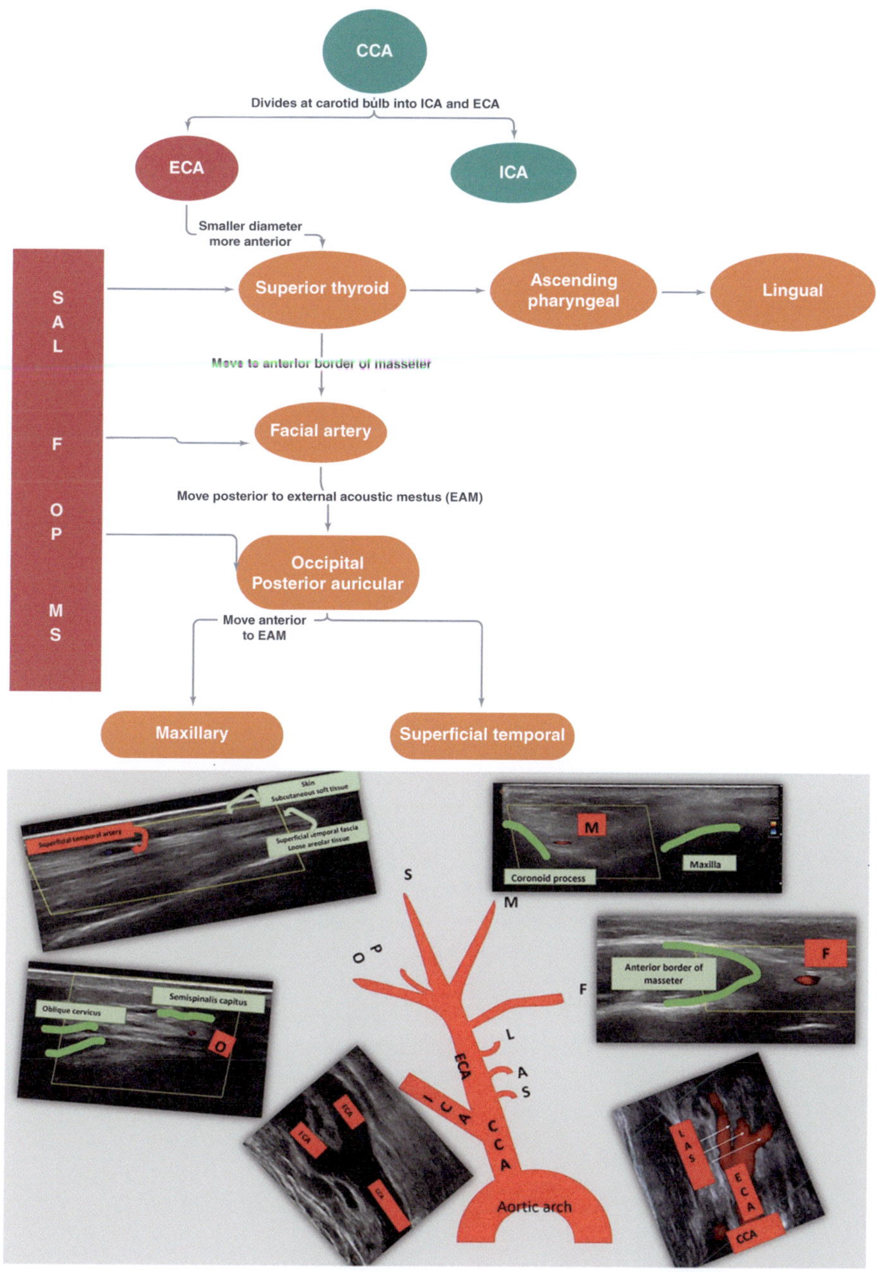

Fig. A.5 External Carotid Artery and its branches

Glossary of Imaging

The glossary includes case studies to further illustrate imaging methods used for aesthetic procedures as well as protocol imaging by various ultrasound manufacturers.

Case Studies

Superficial Temporal Artery VO

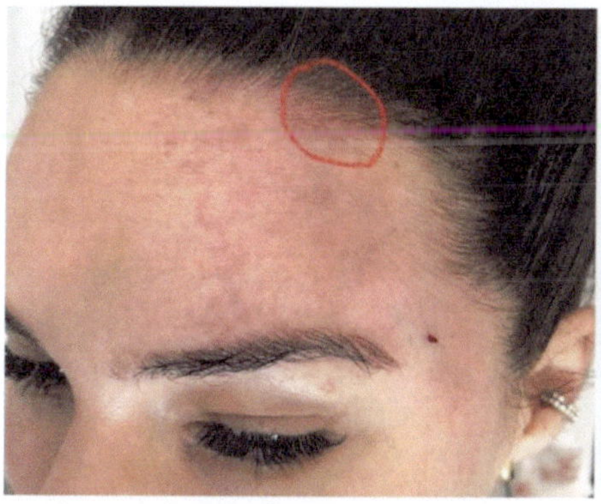

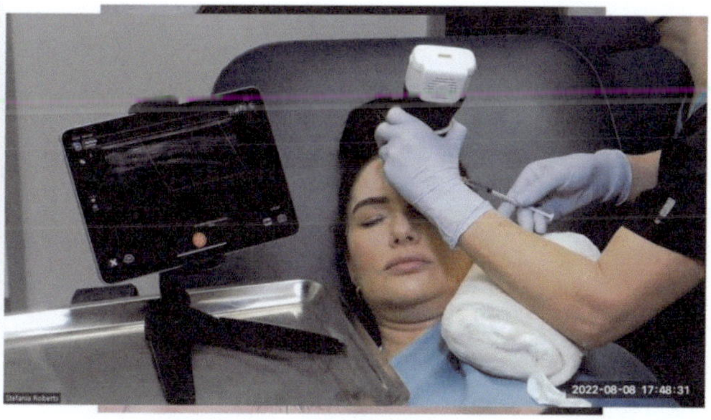

POST Flooding De Lorenzi protocol

Total: 10,500U hyaluronidase

7 days POST
Targeted Ultrasound guided hyaluronidase
Total: 350U hyaluronidase

K. Malherbe, S. Roberts, *Ultrasound Protocol for Facial Aesthetics*,
https://doi.org/10.1007/978-3-031-75949-9

Submental Artery – Targeted Ultrasound Guided Hyaluronidase

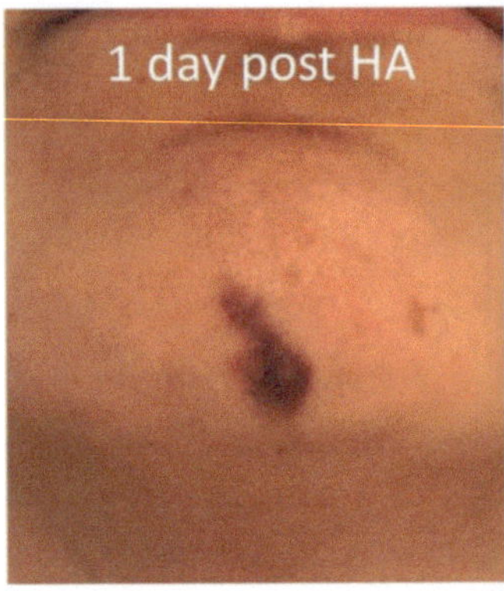

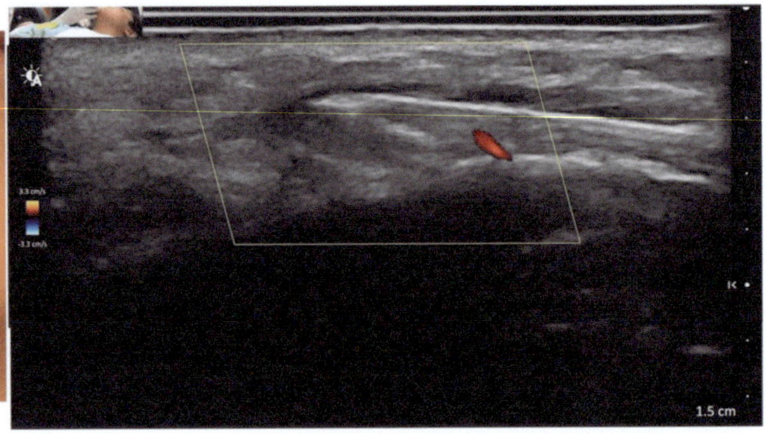

Total:190U hyaluronidase

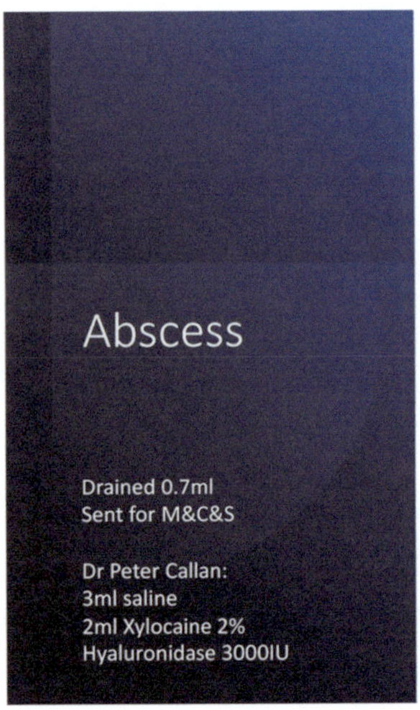

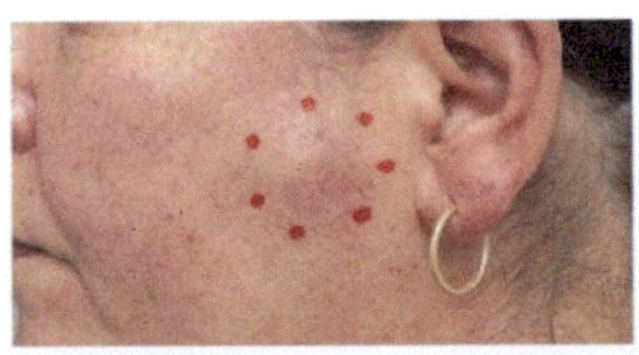

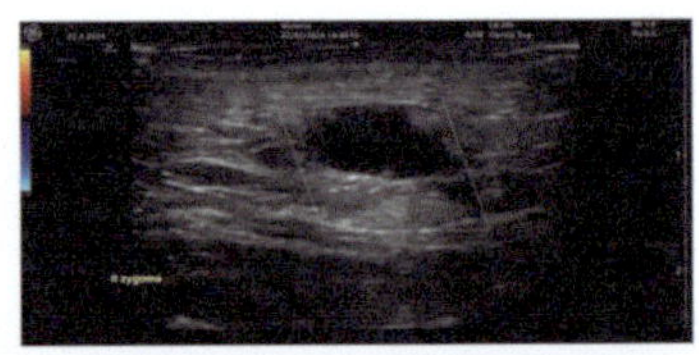

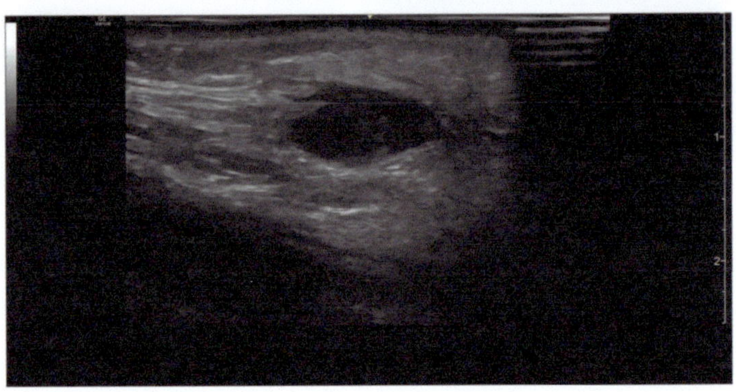

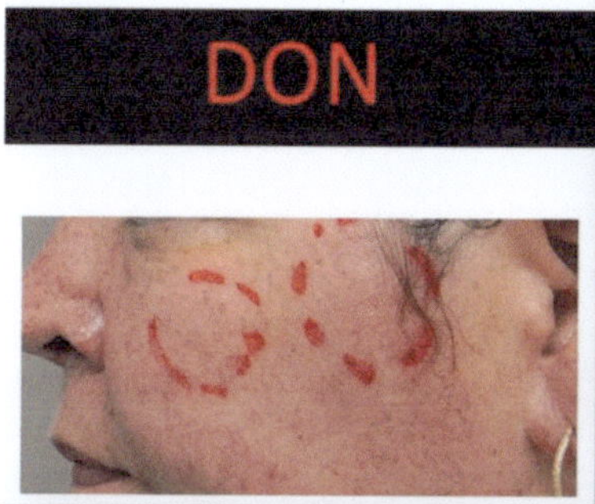

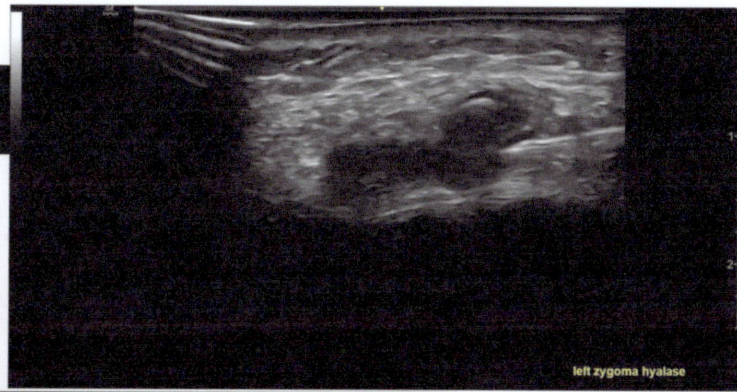

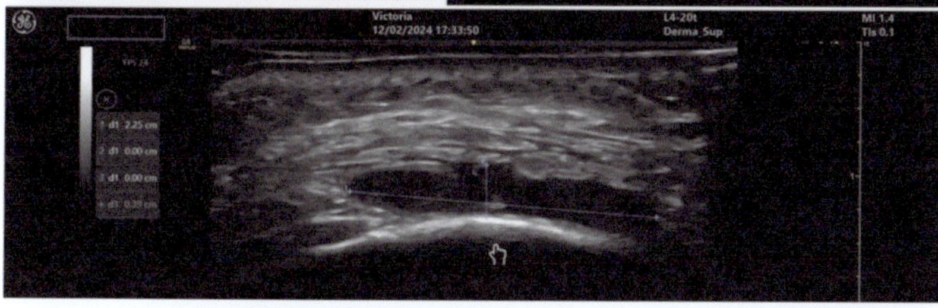

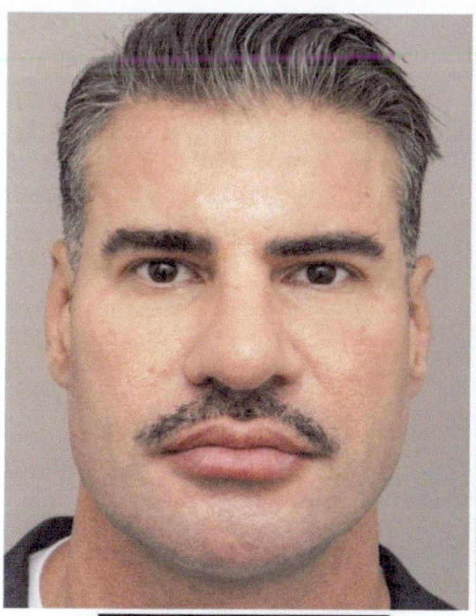

8th February 2024

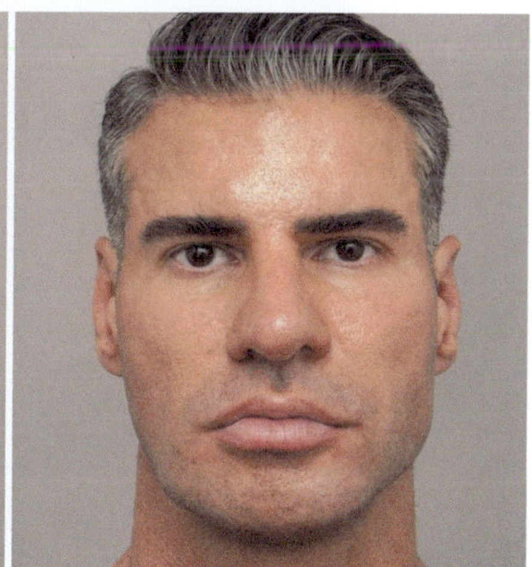

28th February 2024

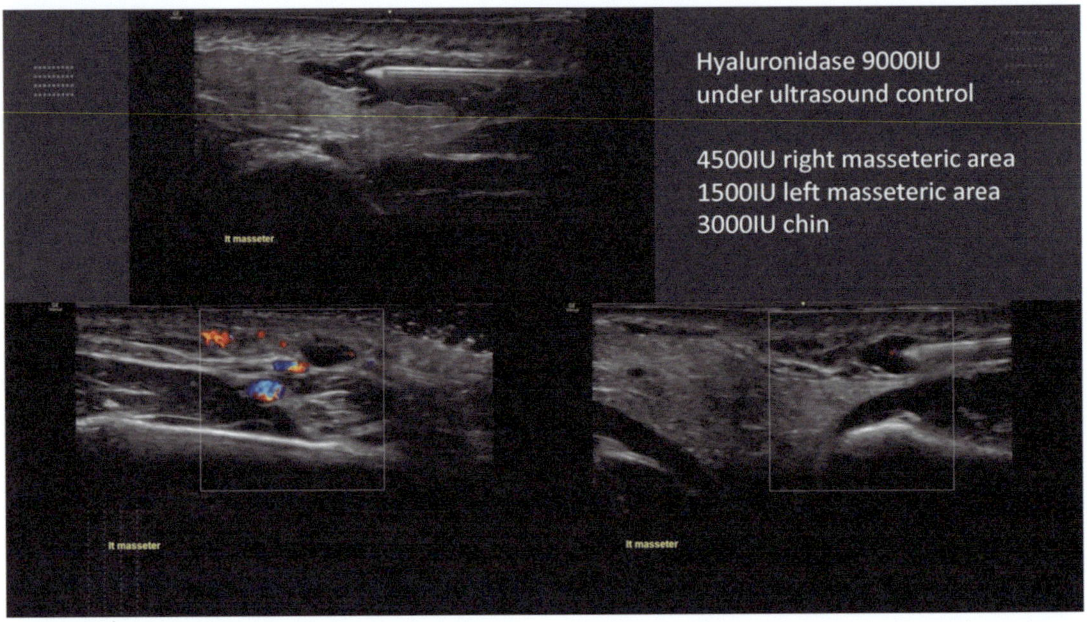
Hyaluronidase 9000IU
under ultrasound control
4500IU right masseteric area
1500IU left masseteric area
3000IU chin
lt masseter
lt masseter
lt masseter

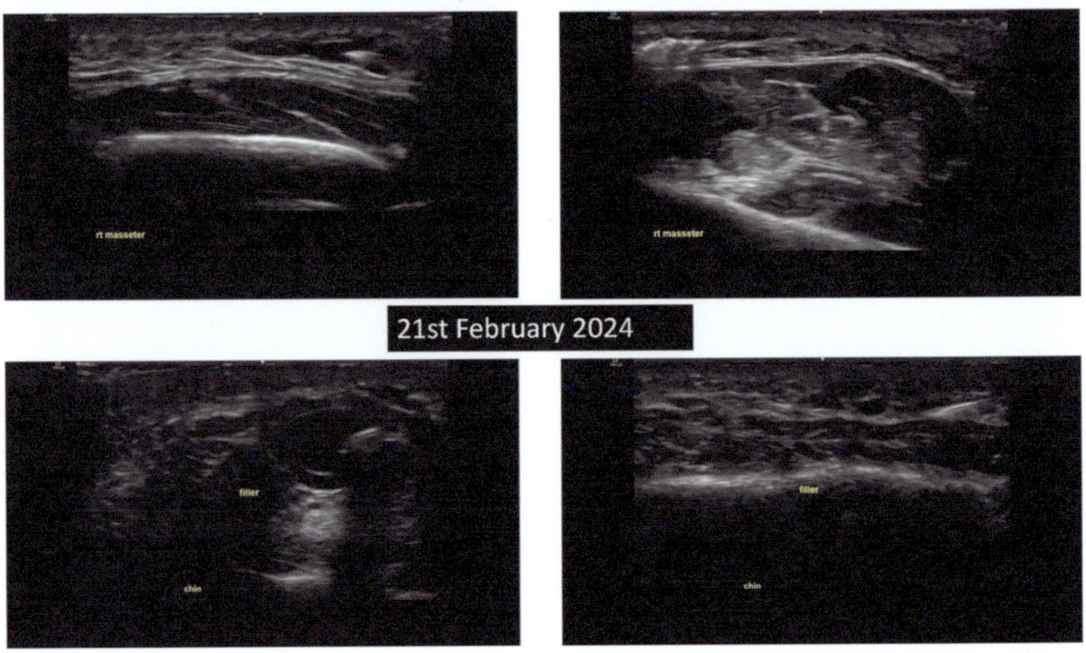
rt masseter
rt masseter
21st February 2024
filler
chin
filler
chin

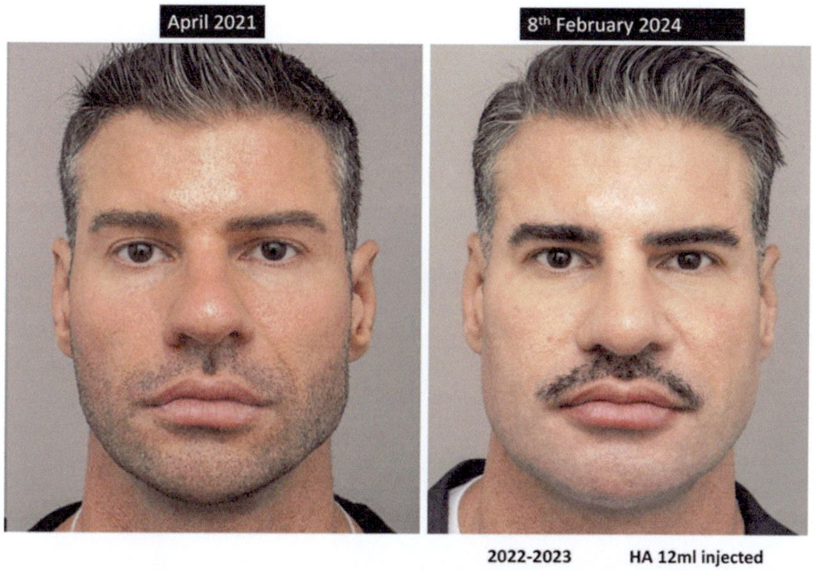
April 2021
8th February 2024
2022-2023
HA 12ml injected

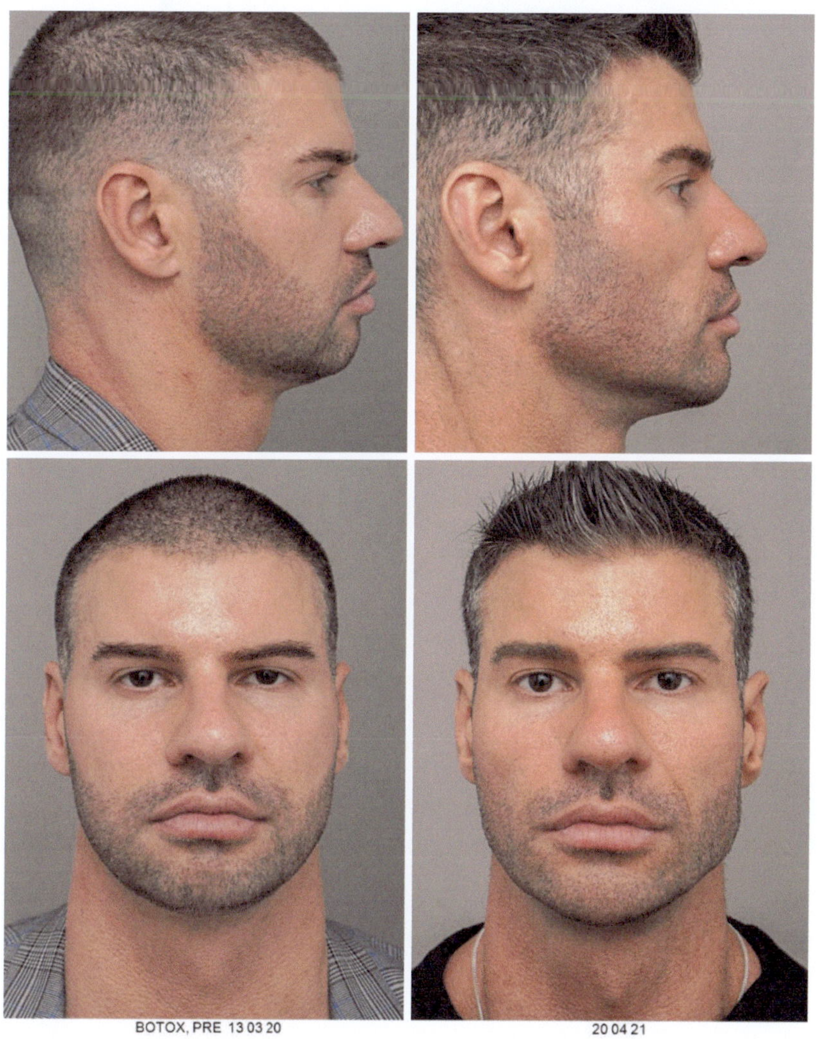
BOTOX, PRE 13 03 20
20 04 21

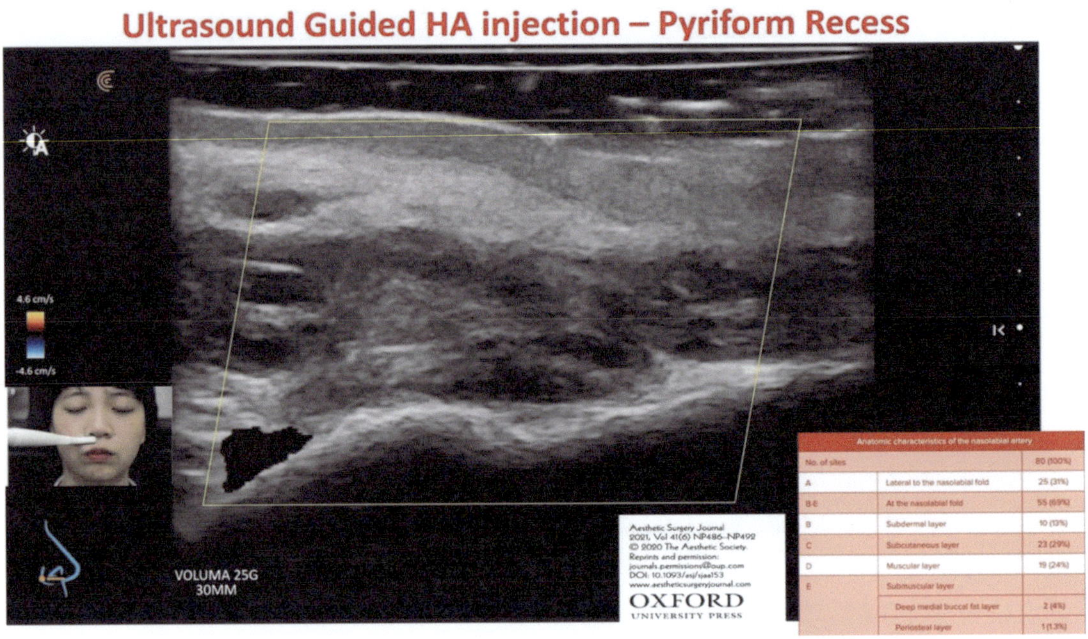
Ultrasound Guided HA injection – Pyriform Recess
4.6 cm/s
-4.6 cm/s
VOLUMA 25G
30MM
Aesthetic Surgery Journal
2021, Vol 41(6) NP486–NP492
© 2020 The Aesthetic Society
Reprints and permission:
journals.permissions@oup.com
DOI: 10.1093/asj/sjaa153
www.aestheticsurgeryjournal.com
OXFORD
UNIVERSITY PRESS
Anatomic characteristics of the nasolabial artery
No. of sites 80 (100%)
A Lateral to the nasolabial fold 25 (31%)
B-E At the nasolabial fold 55 (69%)
B Subdermal layer 10 (13%)
C Subcutaneous layer 23 (29%)
D Muscular layer 19 (24%)
E Submuscular layer
Deep medial buccal fat layer 2 (4%)
Periosteal layer 1 (1.3%)

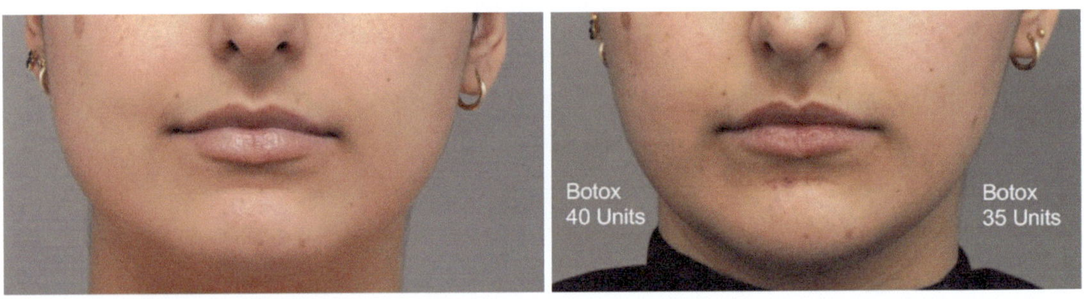
Botox
40 Units
Botox
35 Units

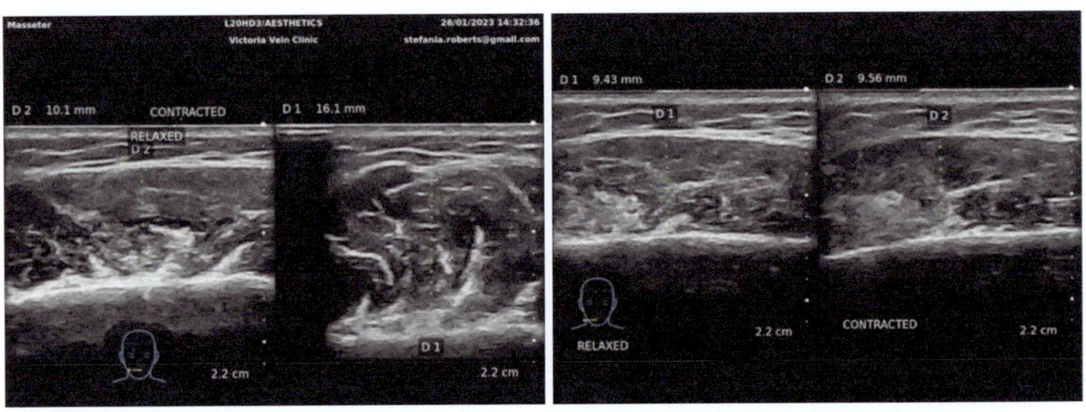
Masseter
L20HD3/AESTHETICS
Victoria Vein Clinic
26/01/2023 14:32:36
stefania.roberts@gmail.com
D 2 10.1 mm
CONTRACTED
D 1 16.1 mm
RELAXED
D 2
D 1
2.2 cm
2.2 cm
D 1 9.43 mm
D 2 9.56 mm
D 1
D 2
RELAXED
2.2 cm
CONTRACTED
2.2 cm

Ultrasound Protocol Imaging

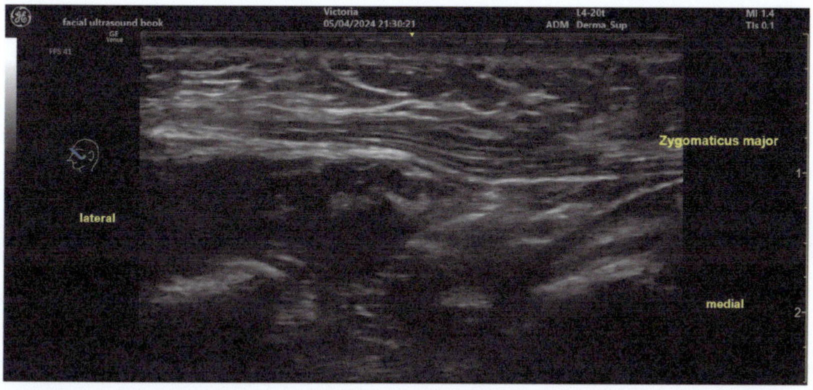

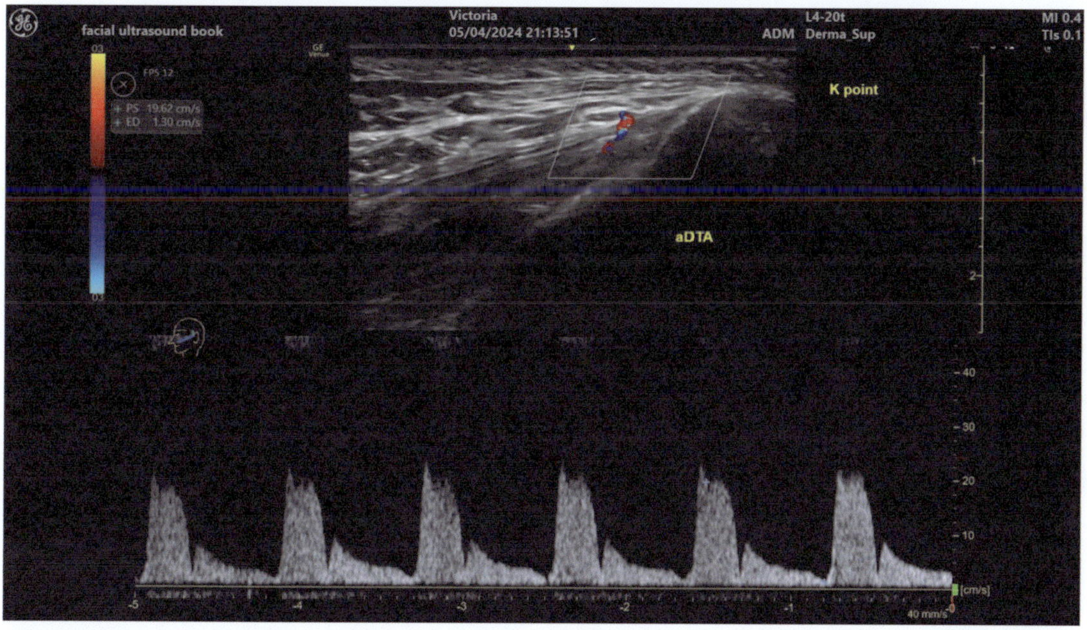

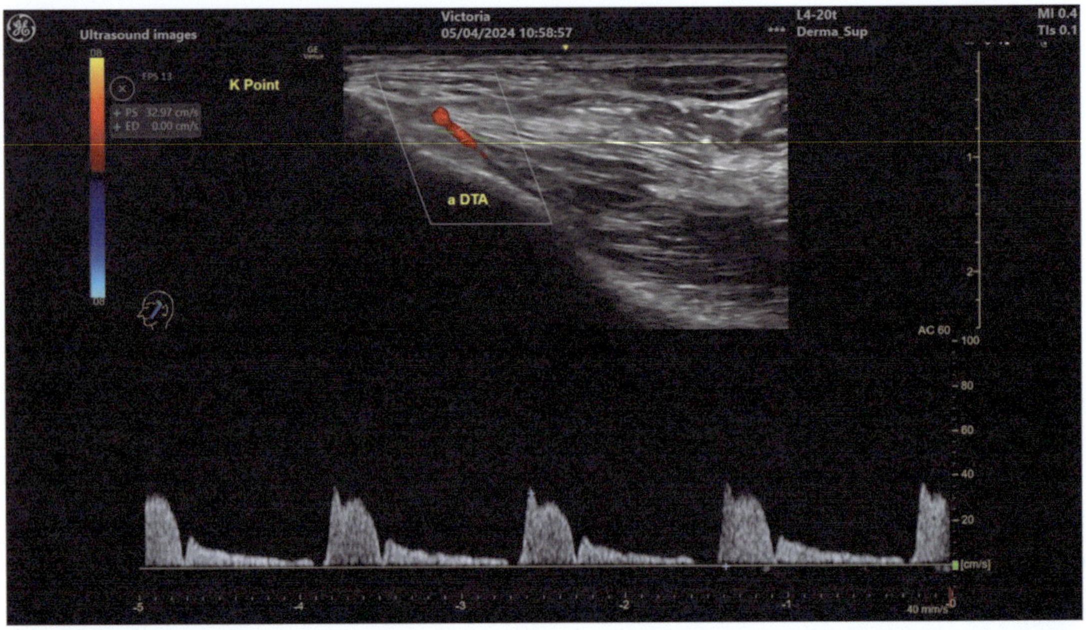
Ultrasound images
Victoria
05/04/2024 10:58:57
L4-20t
Derma_Sup
MI 0.4
TIs 0.1
K Point
a DTA
AC 60
40 mm/s
[cm/s]

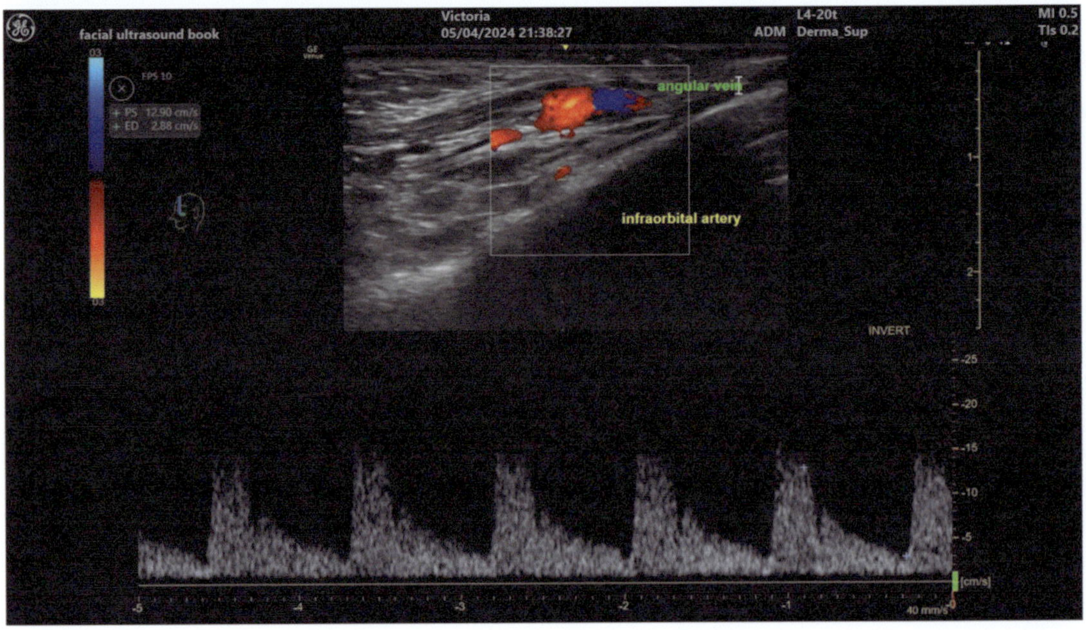
facial ultrasound book
Victoria
05/04/2024 21:38:27
ADM
L4-20t
Derma_Sup
MI 0.5
TIs 0.2
angular vein
infraorbital artery
INVERT
40 mm/s
[cm/s]

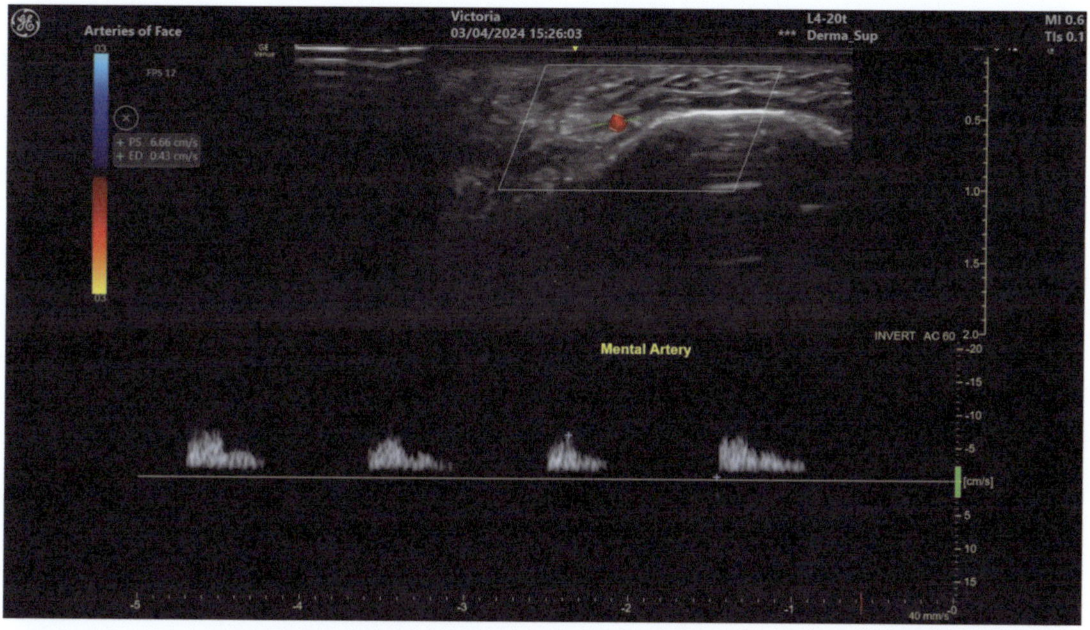
Arteries of Face
Victoria
03/04/2024 15:26:03
L4-20t
Derma_Sup
MI 0.6
TIs 0.1
FPS 12
PS 6.66 cm/s
ED 0.43 cm/s
Mental Artery
INVERT AC 60
[cm/s]
40 mm/s

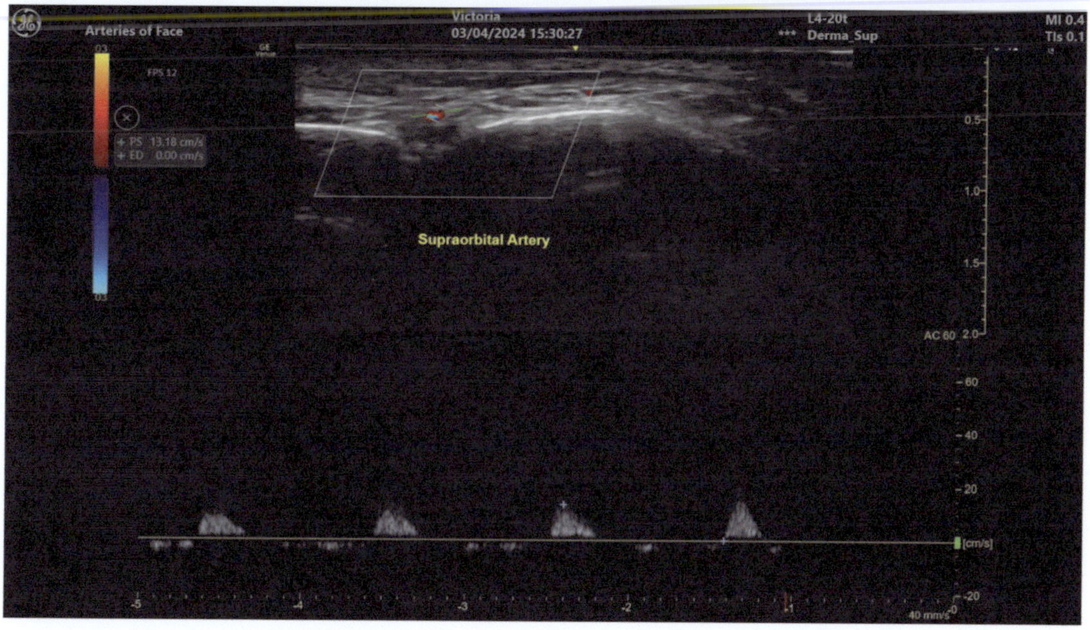
Arteries of Face
Victoria
03/04/2024 15:30:27
L4-20t
Derma_Sup
MI 0.4
TIs 0.1
FPS 12
PS 13.18 cm/s
ED 0.00 cm/s
Supraorbital Artery
AC 60
[cm/s]
40 mm/s

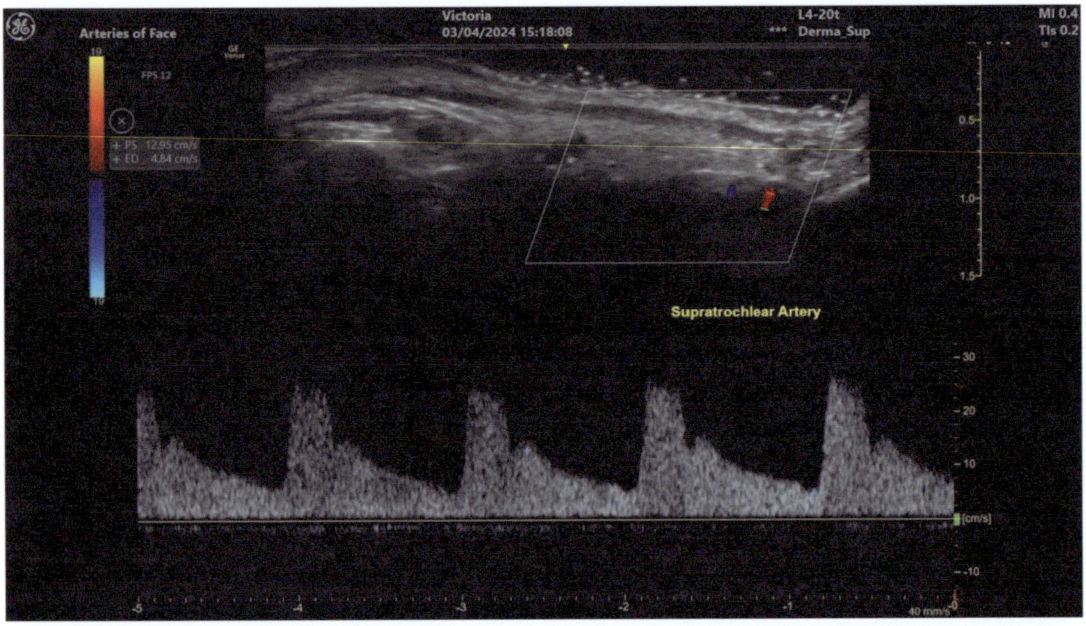
Arteries of Face
Victoria
03/04/2024 15:18:08
L4-20t
*** Derma_Sup
MI 0.4
TIs 0.2
Supratrochlear Artery

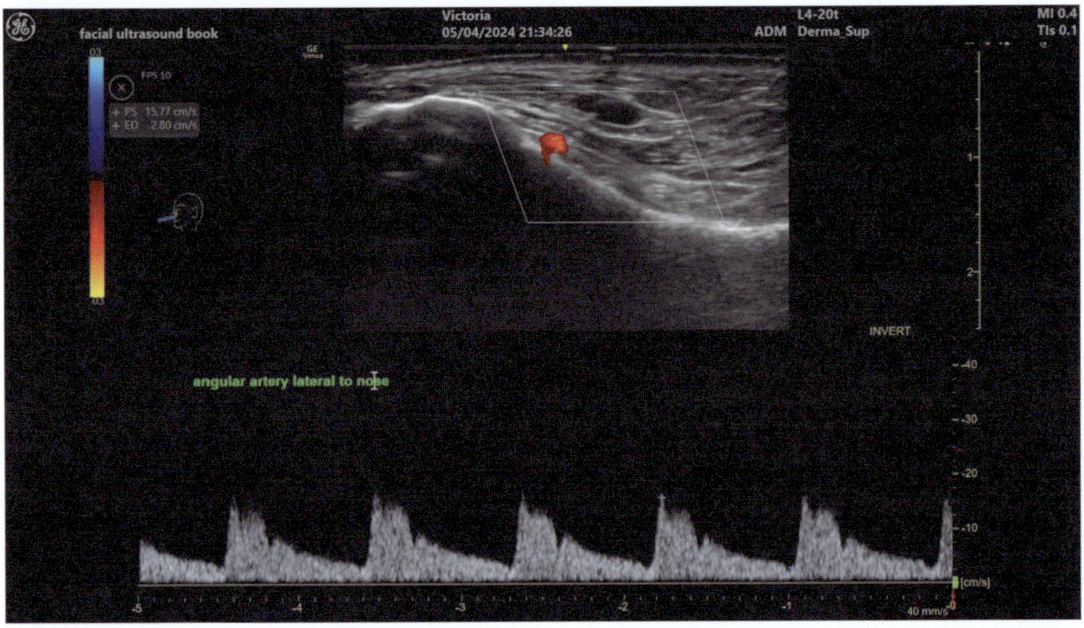
facial ultrasound book
Victoria
05/04/2024 21:34:26
L4-20t
ADM Derma_Sup
MI 0.4
TIs 0.1
INVERT
angular artery lateral to nose

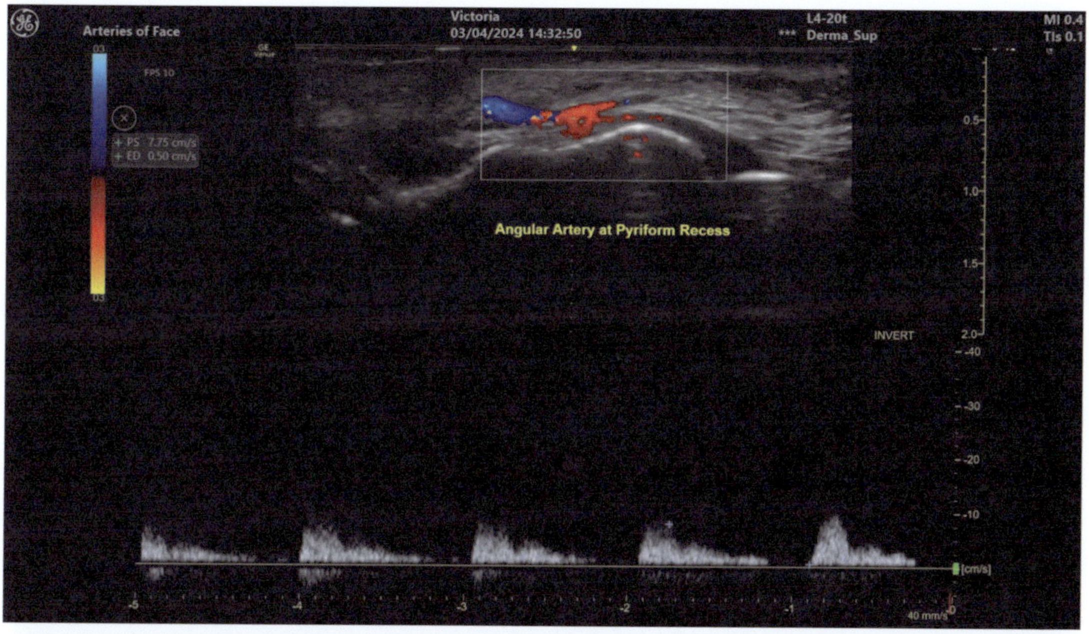
Arteries of Face
Victoria
03/04/2024 14:32:50
L4-20t
Derma_Sup
MI 0.4
TIs 0.1
PS 7.75 cm/s
ED 0.50 cm/s
Angular Artery at Pyriform Recess
INVERT
[cm/s]
40 mm/s

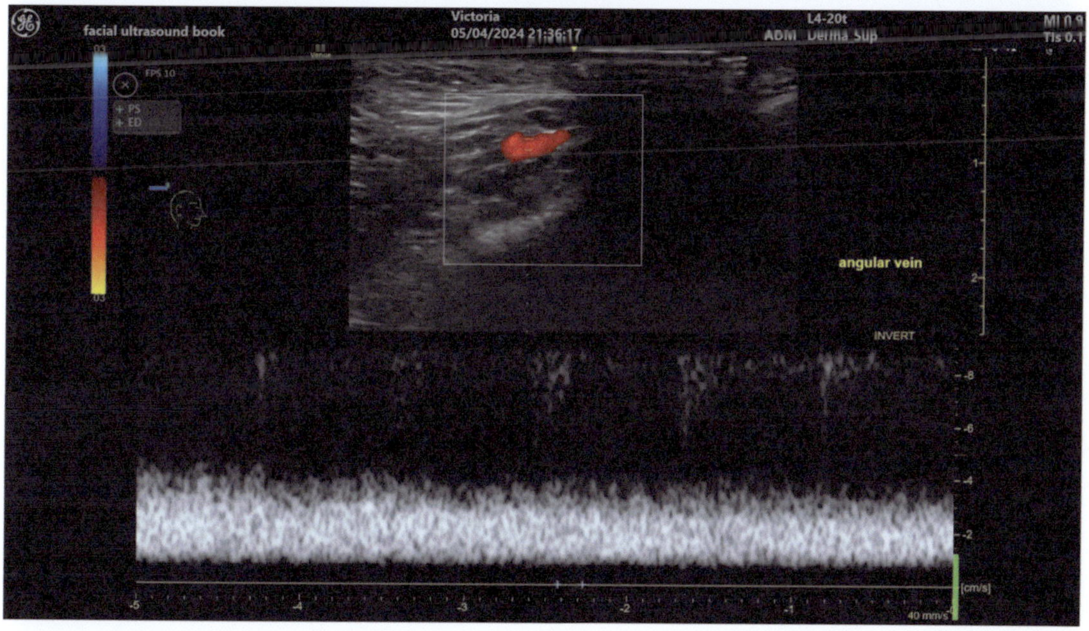
facial ultrasound book
Victoria
05/04/2024 21:36:17
L4-20t
Derma_Sup
MI 0.9
TIs 0.1
angular vein
INVERT
[cm/s]
40 mm/s

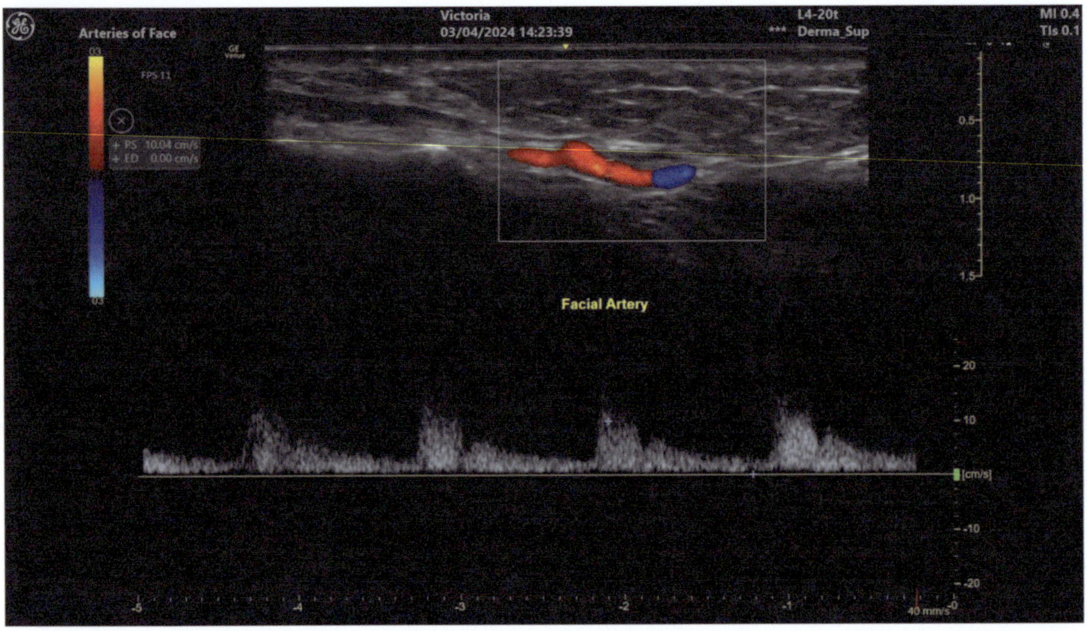
Arteries of Face
Victoria
03/04/2024 14:23:39
L4-20t
*** Derma_Sup
MI 0.4
TIs 0.1
FPS 11
PS 10.04 cm/s
ED 0.00 cm/s
Facial Artery
[cm/s]
40 mm/s

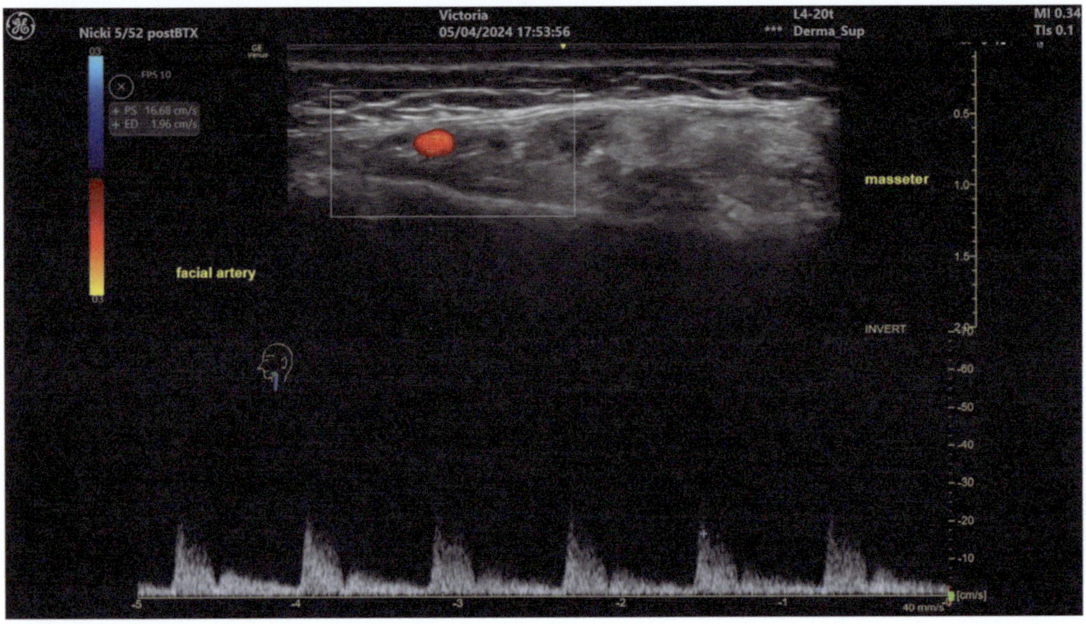
Nicki 5/52 postBTX
Victoria
05/04/2024 17:53:56
L4-20t
*** Derma_Sup
MI 0.34
TIs 0.1
FPS 10
PS 16.68 cm/s
ED 1.96 cm/s
masseter
facial artery
INVERT
[cm/s]
40 mm/s

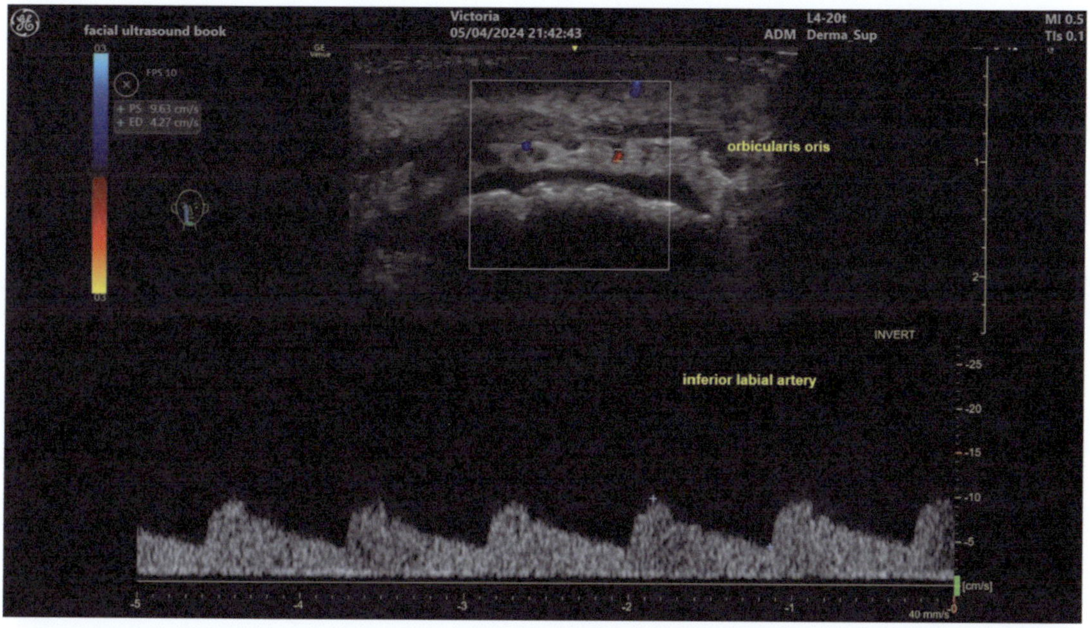
Victoria
05/04/2024 21:42:43
facial ultrasound book
L4-20t
ADM Derma_Sup
MI 0.5
TIs 0.1
orbicularis oris
INVERT
inferior labial artery
[cm/s]
40 mm/s

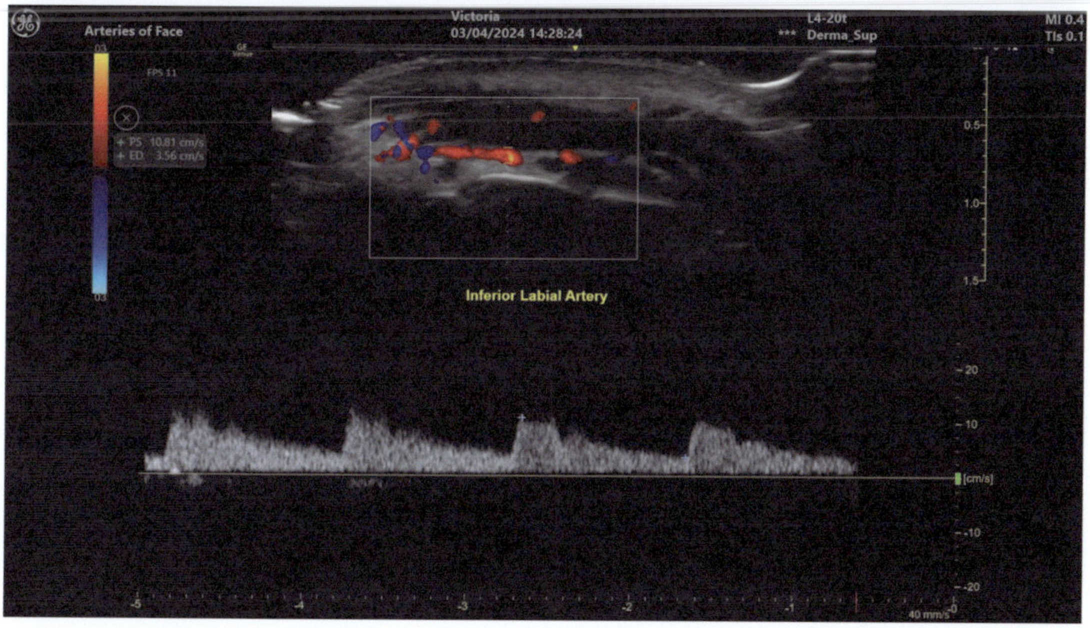
Victoria
03/04/2024 14:28:24
Arteries of Face
L4-20t
Derma_Sup
MI 0.4
TIs 0.1
Inferior Labial Artery
[cm/s]
40 mm/s

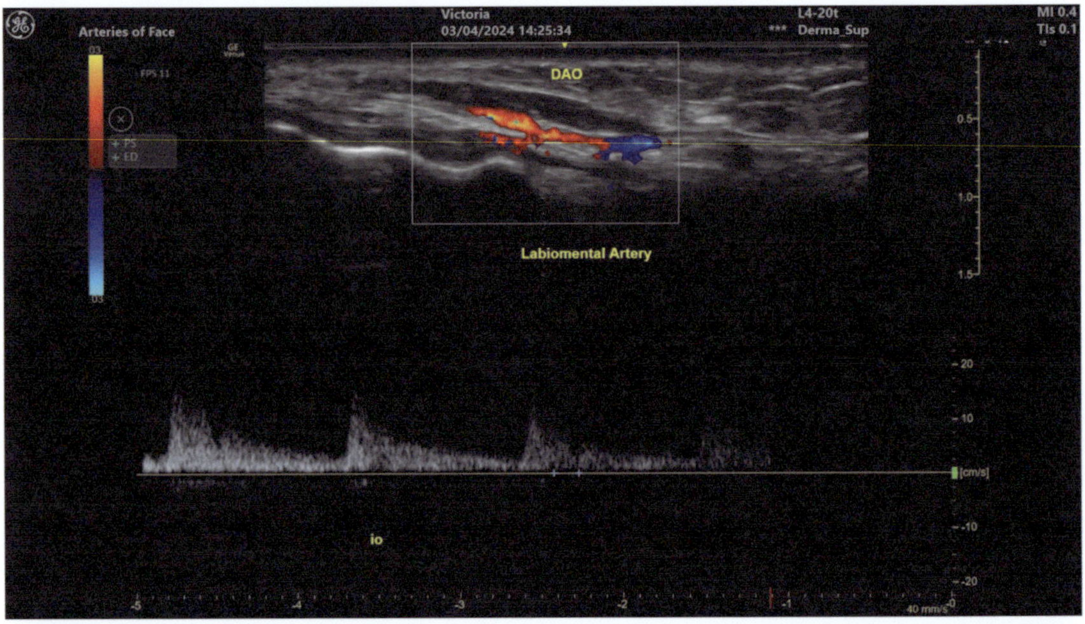
Victoria
03/04/2024 14:25:34
L4-20t
*** Derma_Sup
MI 0.4
TIs 0.1
Arteries of Face
DAO
Labiomental Artery
io
[cm/s]
40 mm/s

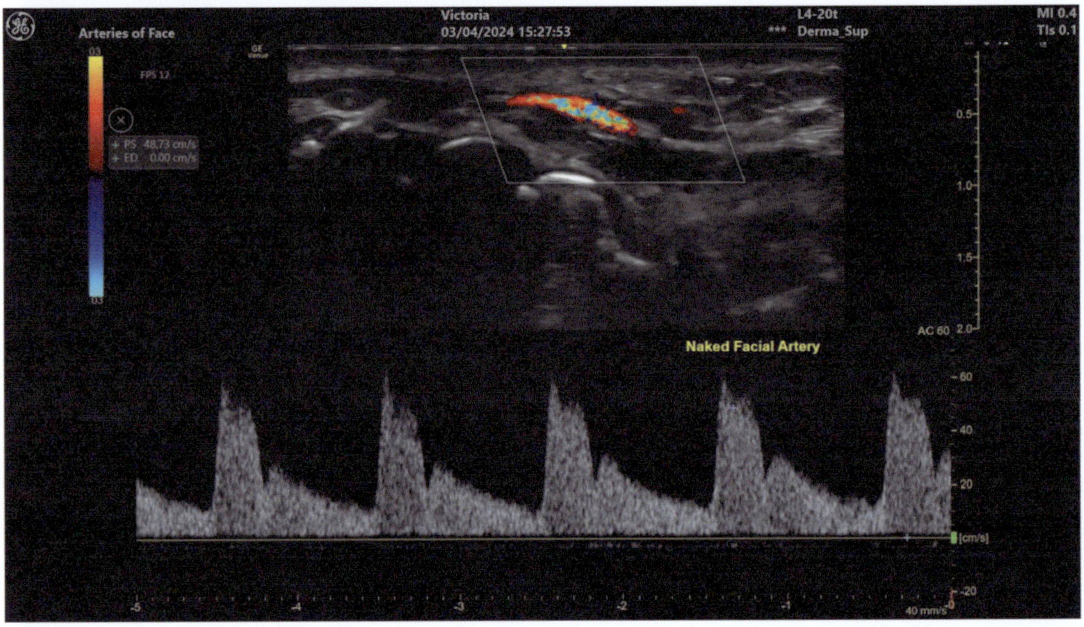
Victoria
03/04/2024 15:27:53
L4-20t
*** Derma_Sup
MI 0.4
TIs 0.1
Arteries of Face
PS 48.73 cm/s
ED 0.00 cm/s
Naked Facial Artery
AC 60
[cm/s]
40 mm/s

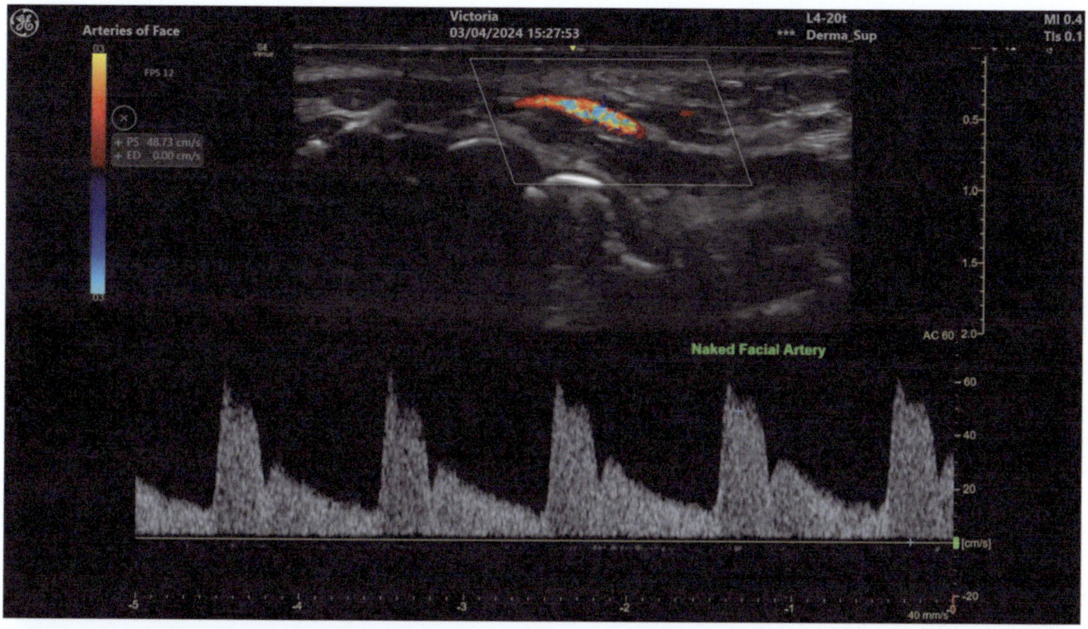
Arteries of Face
Victoria
03/04/2024 15:27:53
L4-20t
Derma_Sup
MI 0.4
TIs 0.1
PS 48.73 cm/s
ED 0.00 cm/s
Naked Facial Artery
[cm/s]
40 mm/s

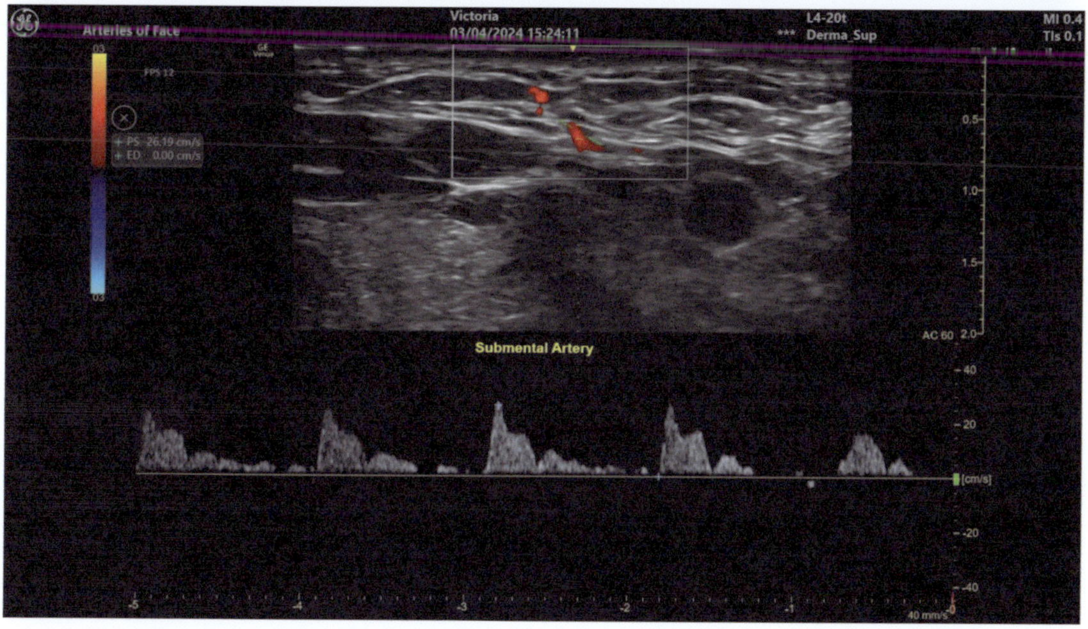
Arteries of Face
Victoria
03/04/2024 15:24:11
L4-20t
Derma_Sup
MI 0.4
TIs 0.1
PS 26.19 cm/s
ED 0.00 cm/s
Submental Artery
[cm/s]
40 mm/s

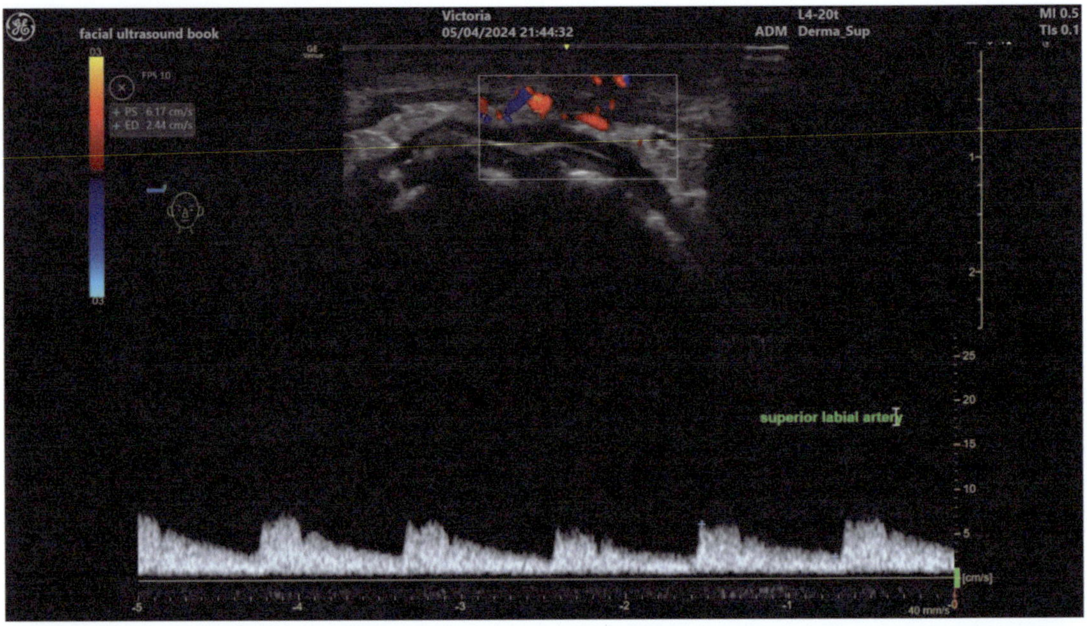
facial ultrasound book
Victoria
05/04/2024 21:44:32
L4-20t
ADM Derma_Sup
MI 0.5
TIs 0.1
superior labial artery
[cm/s]
40 mm/s

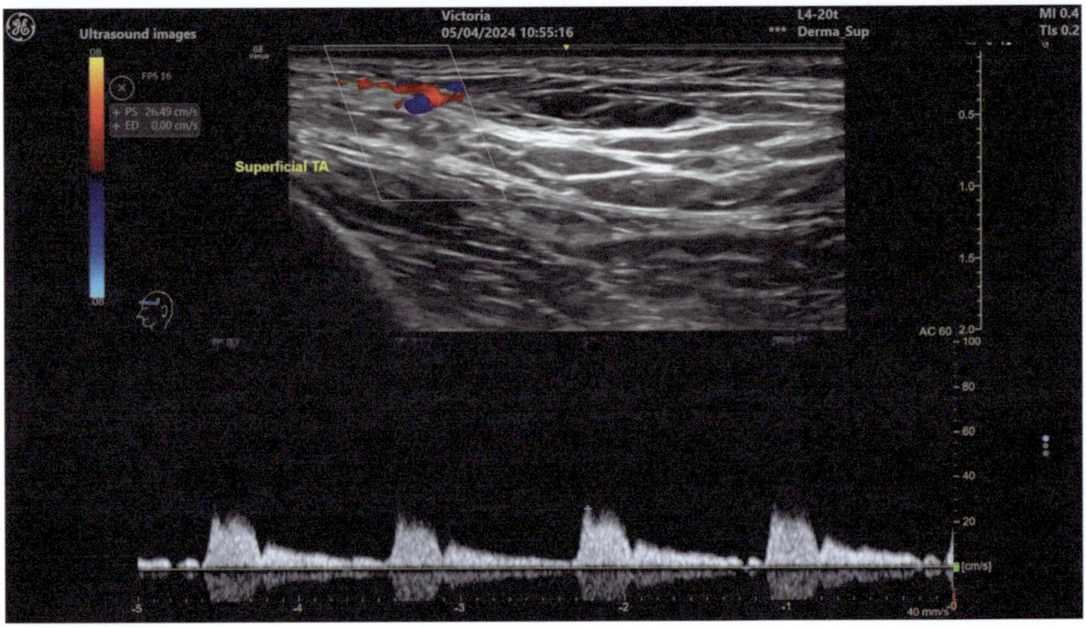
Ultrasound images
Victoria
05/04/2024 10:55:16
L4-20t
Derma_Sup
MI 0.4
TIs 0.2
Superficial TA
AC 60
[cm/s]
40 mm/s

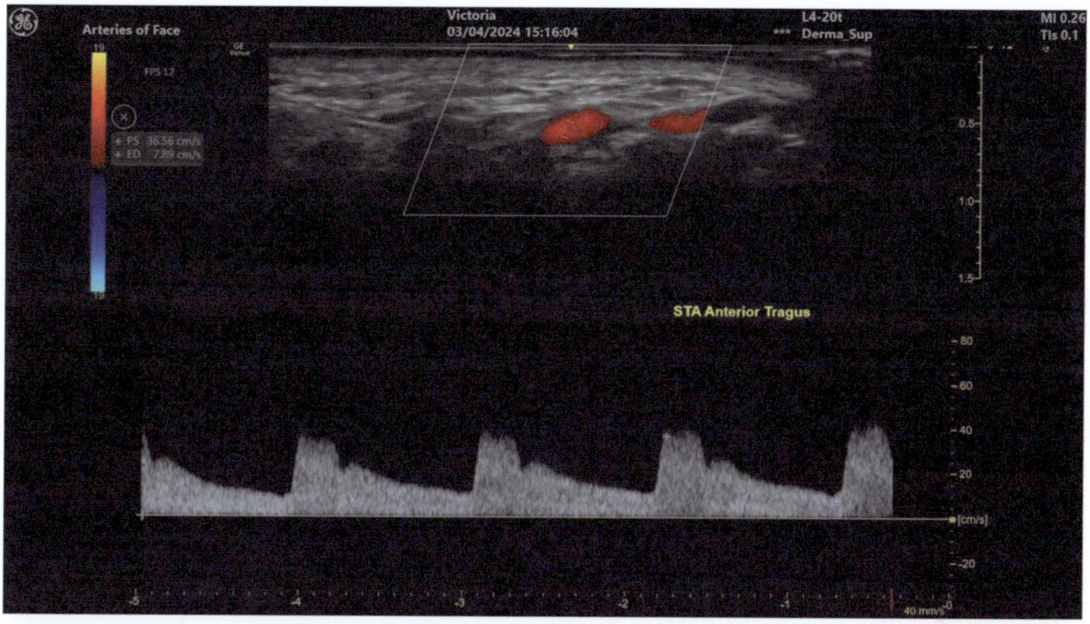
Arteries of Face
Victoria
03/04/2024 15:16:04
L4-20t
*** Derma_Sup
MI 0.26
TIs 0.1
PS 36.56 cm/s
ED 7.89 cm/s
STA Anterior Tragus
[cm/s]
40 mm/s

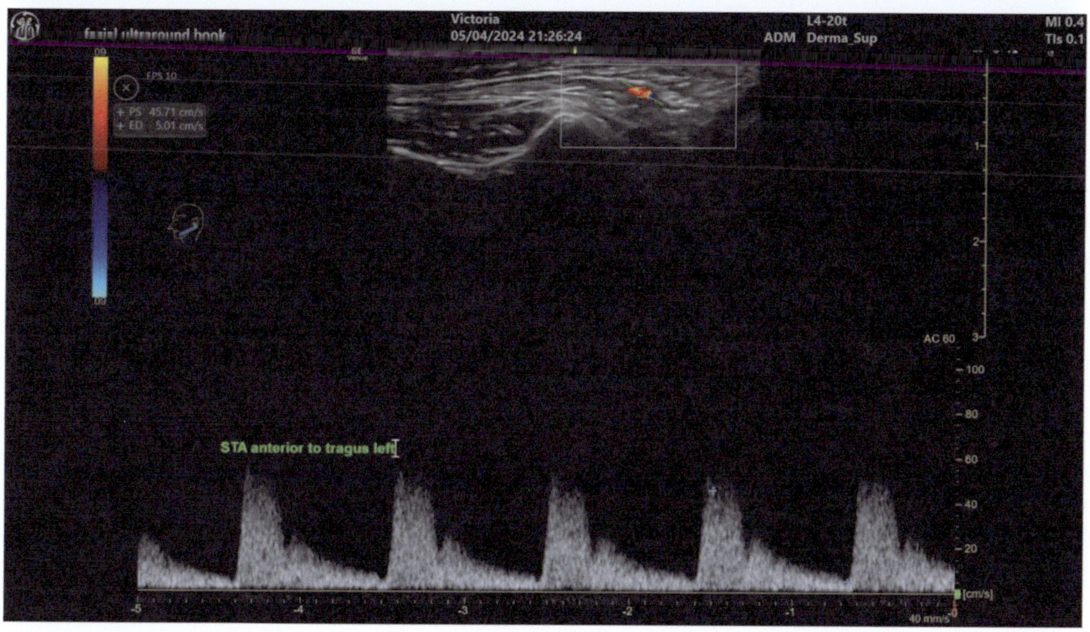
fazial ultrasound book
Victoria
05/04/2024 21:26:24
L4-20t
ADM Derma_Sup
MI 0.4
TIs 0.1
PS 45.71 cm/s
ED 5.01 cm/s
AC 60
STA anterior to tragus left
[cm/s]
40 mm/s

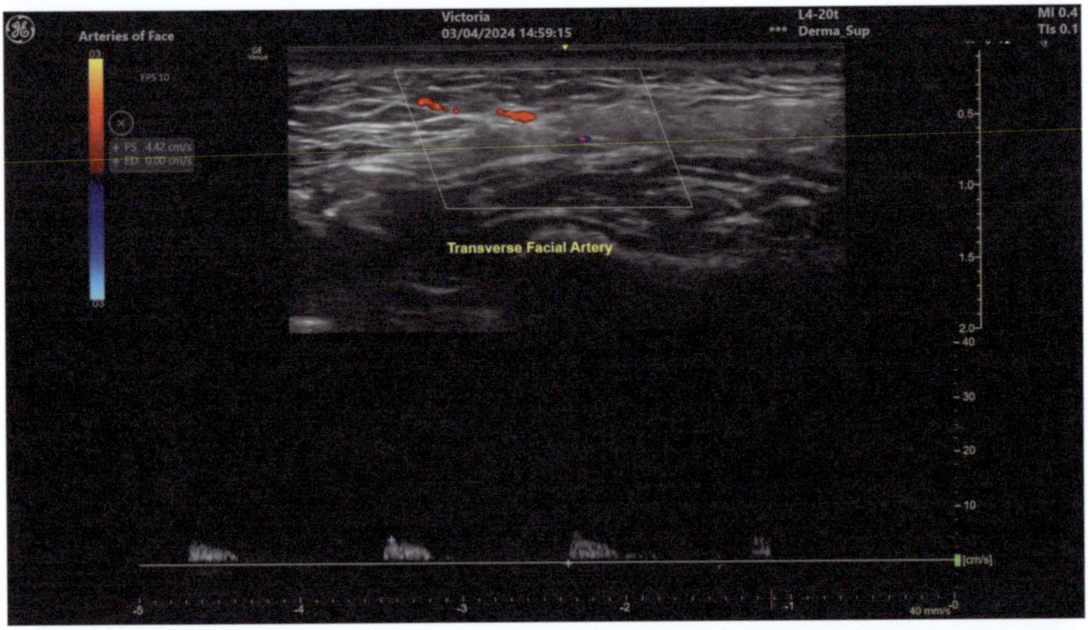
Arteries of Face
Victoria
03/04/2024 14:59:15
L4-20t
Derma_Sup
MI 0.4
TIs 0.1
FPS 10
Transverse Facial Artery
[cm/s]
40 mm/s

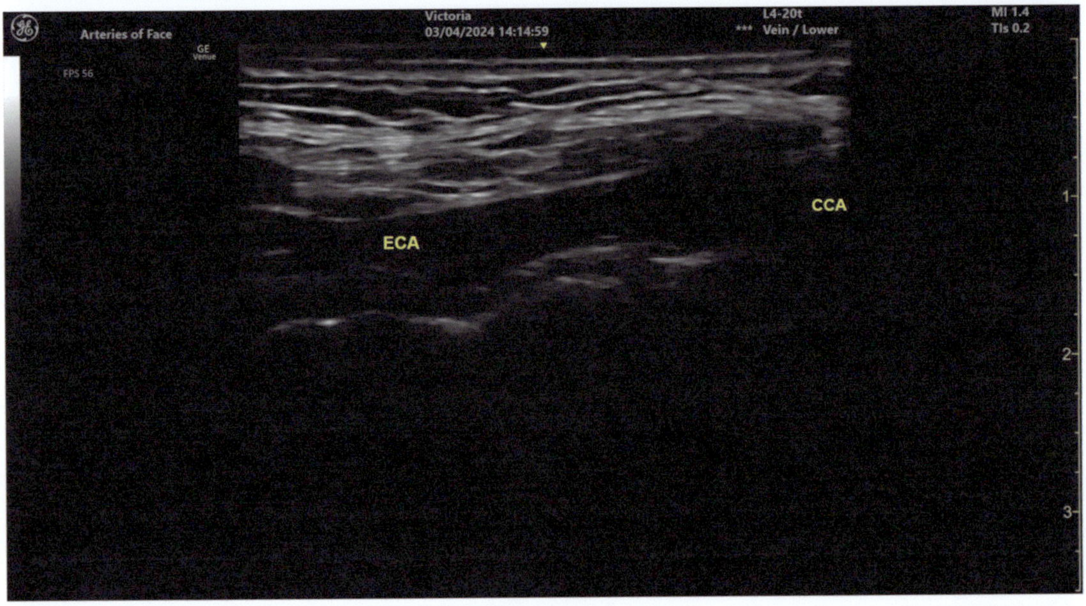
Arteries of Face
Victoria
03/04/2024 14:14:59
L4-20t
Vein / Lower
MI 1.4
TIs 0.2
FPS 56
ECA
CCA

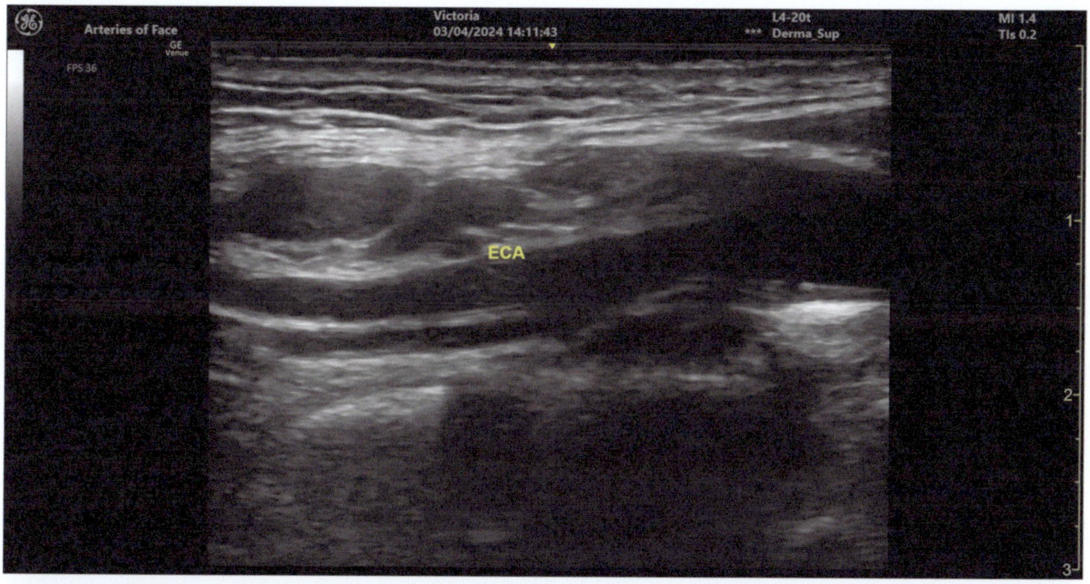

Arteries of Face
Victoria
03/04/2024 14:11:43
L4-20t
Derma_Sup
MI 1.4
TIs 0.2
ECA

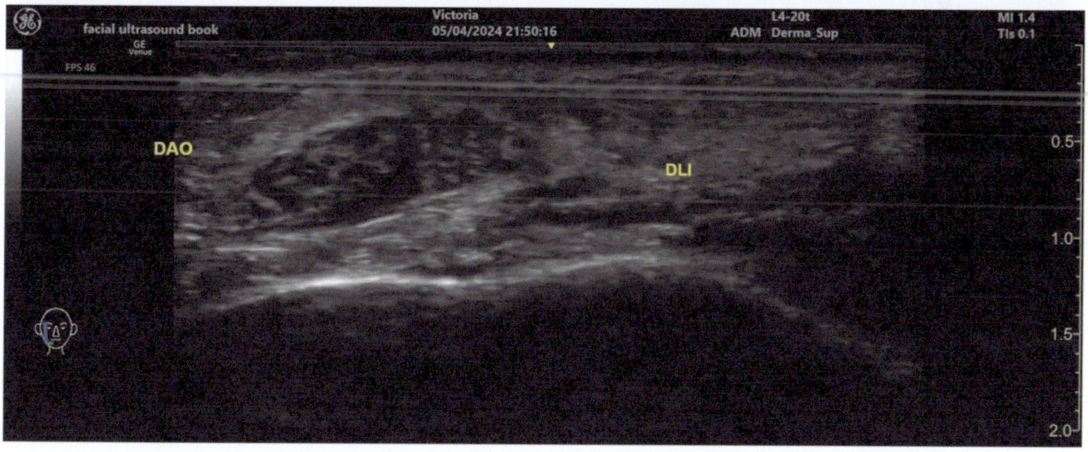

facial ultrasound book
Victoria
05/04/2024 21:50:16
L4-20t
ADM Derma_Sup
MI 1.4
TIs 0.1
DAO
DLI

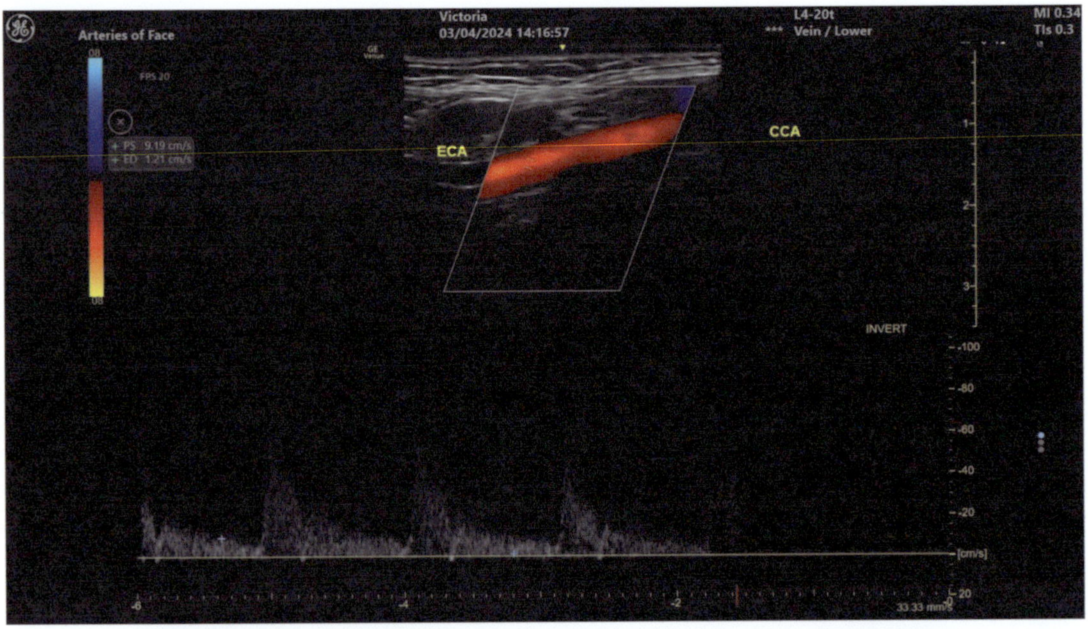
Arteries of Face
Victoria
03/04/2024 14:16:57
L4-20t
*** Vein / Lower
MI 0.34
TIs 0.3
FPS 20
+ PS 9.19 cm/s
+ ED 1.21 cm/s
ECA
CCA
INVERT
[cm/s]
33.33 mm/s

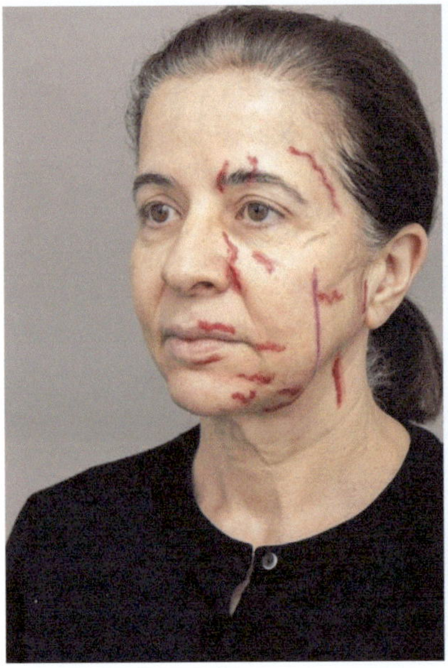

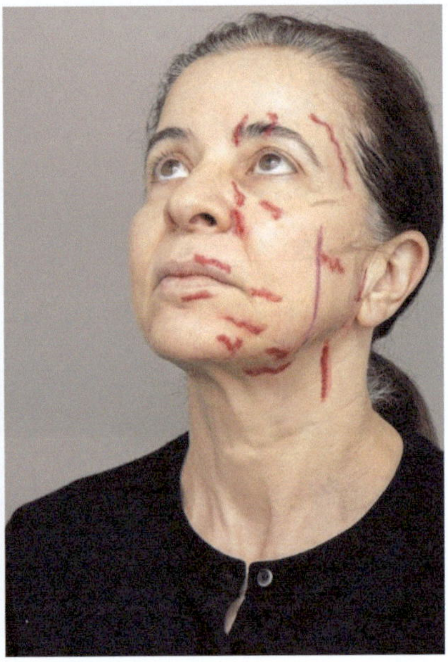

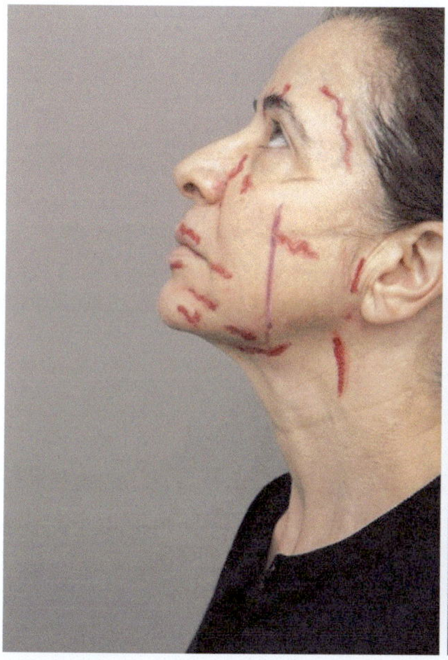

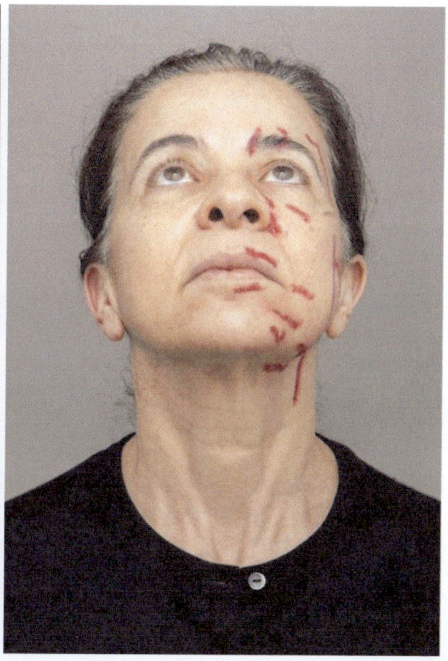

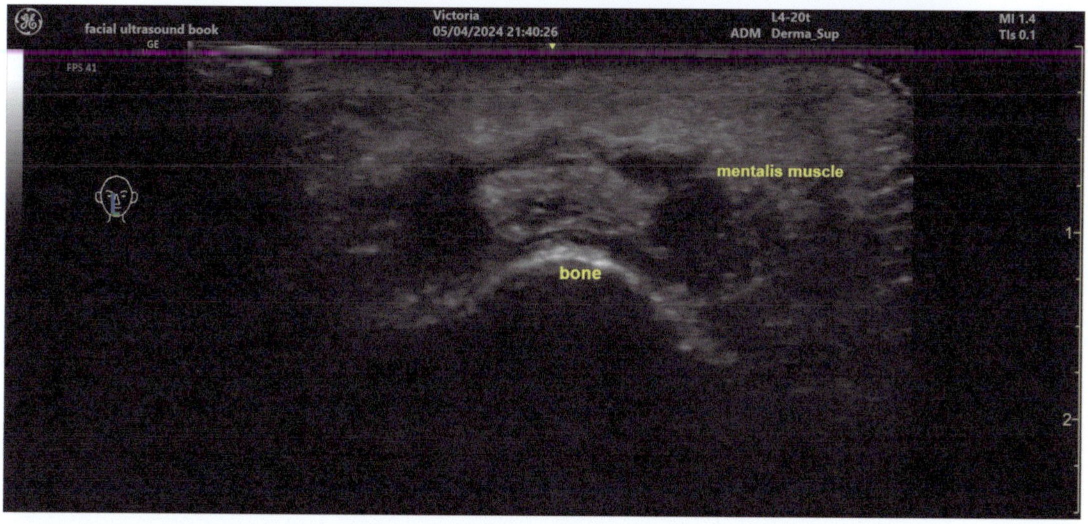
facial ultrasound book
Victoria
05/04/2024 21:40:26
L4-20t
ADM Derma_Sup
MI 1.4
TIs 0.1
mentalis muscle
bone
1
2

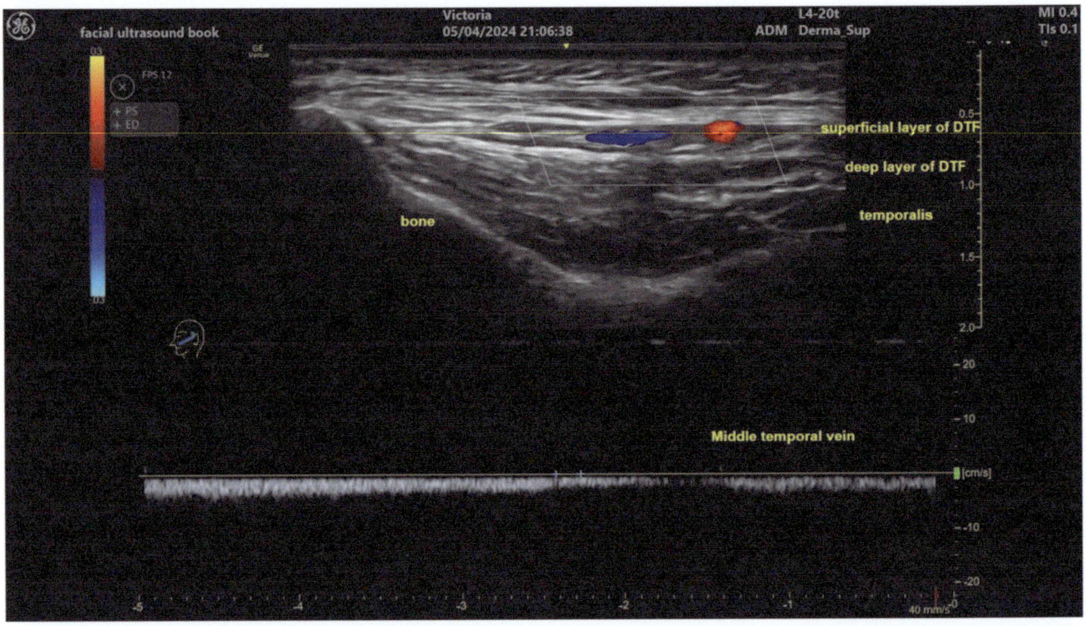
facial ultrasound book
Victoria
05/04/2024 21:06:38
L4-20t
ADM Derma_Sup
MI 0.4
TIs 0.1
superficial layer of DTF
deep layer of DTF
temporalis
bone
Middle temporal vein

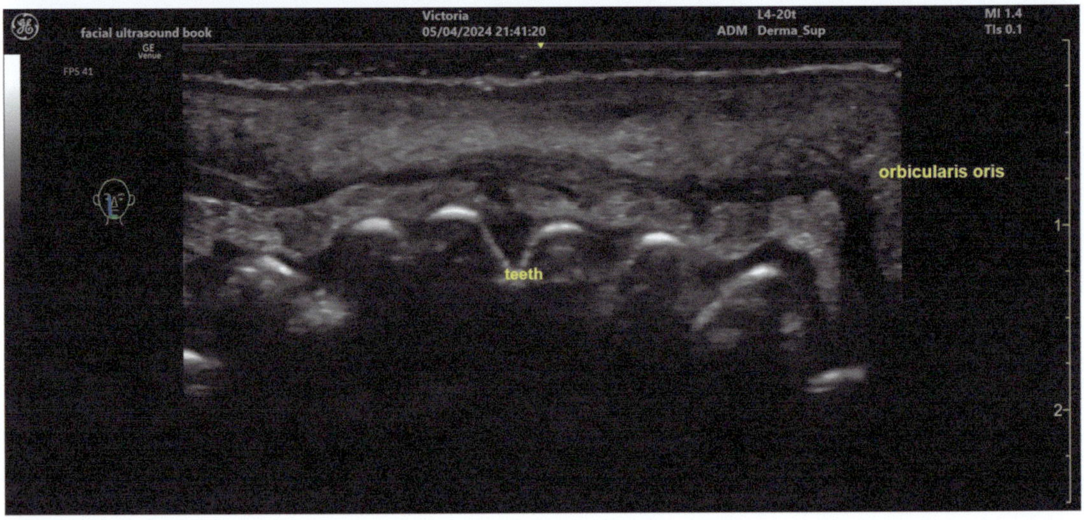
facial ultrasound book
Victoria
05/04/2024 21:41:20
L4-20t
ADM Derma_Sup
MI 1.4
TIs 0.1
orbicularis oris
teeth

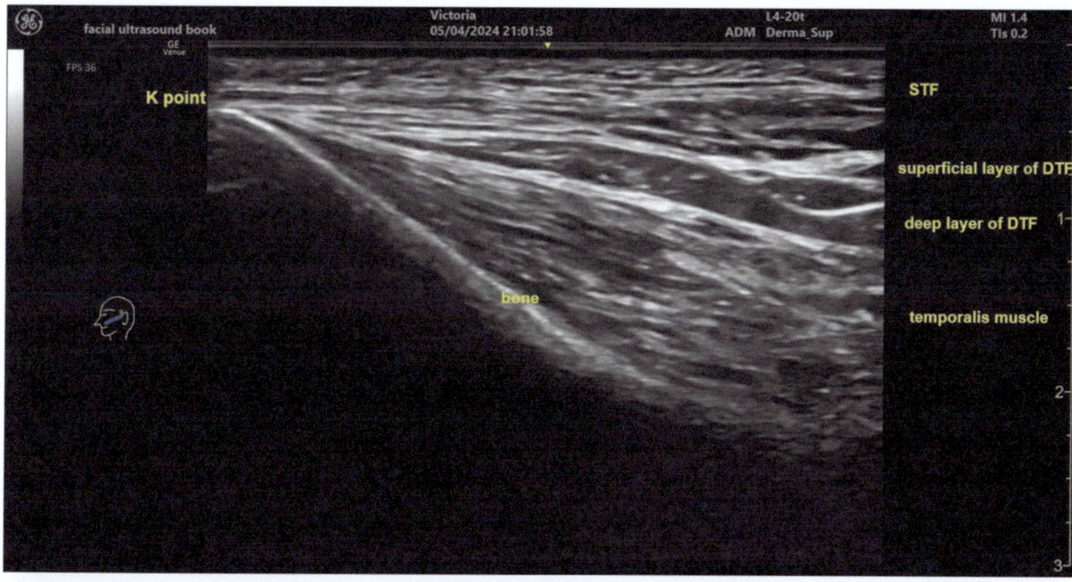

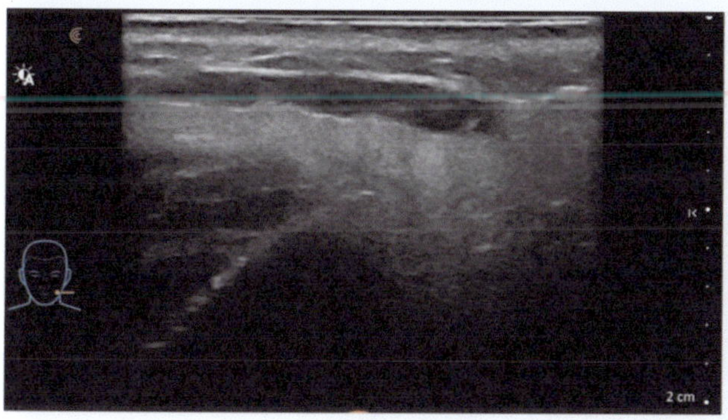

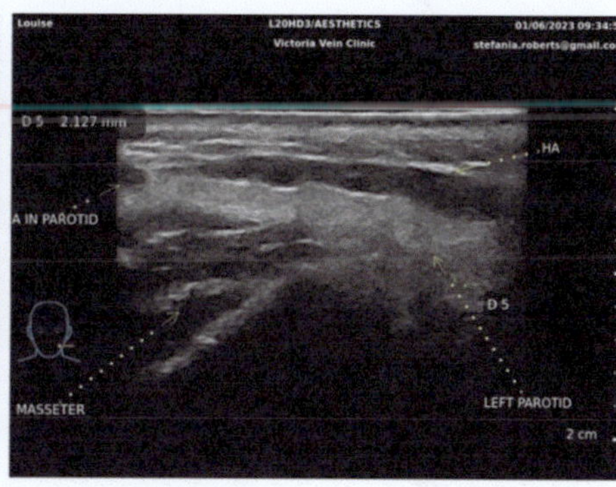

Ultrasound Guided Hyaluronidase –
Intraparotid HA

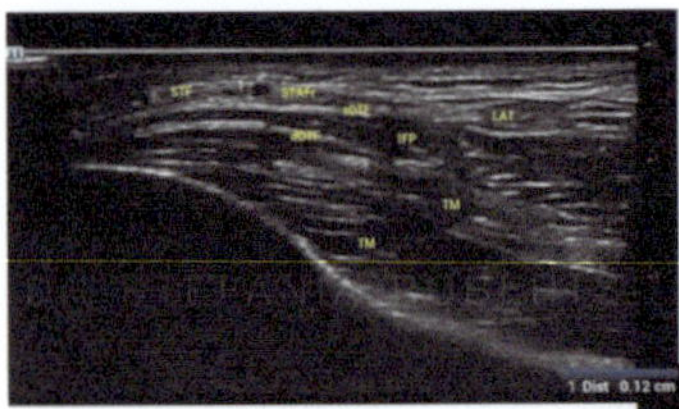

Ultrasound Guided HA injection – Temporal Fossa

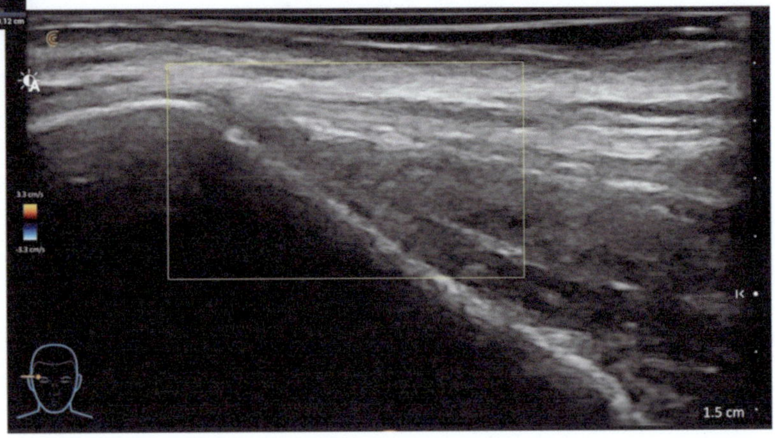

ULTRASOUND MORPHOLOGY OF SILICONE OIL

ULTRASOUND MORPHOLOGY OF POLYMETHYLMETHACRYLATE - PMMA

MATRIX WITH HYPERECHOIC DEPOSITS WITH HYPERECHOIC AREAS

MINI COMET TAIL ARTIFACT

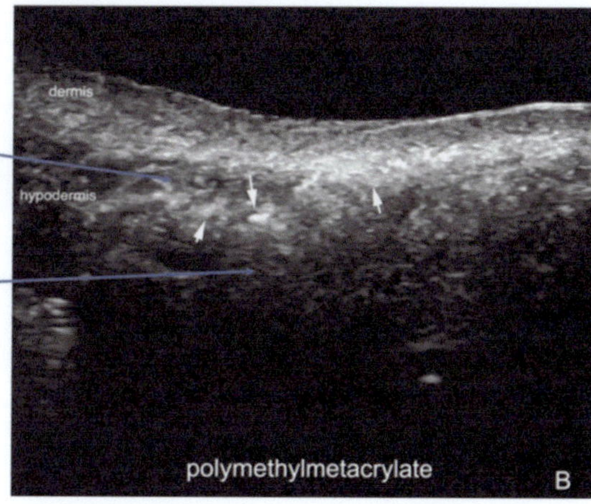

Ultrasound Morphology of Polycaprolactone Filler

Ximena Wortsman, MD, Natacha Quezada, MD

 | J Ultrasound Med 2017; 00:00–00 | 0278-4297 | www.aium.org

ULTRASOUND MORPHOLOGY OF POLYCAPROLACTONE (PLA)

MATRIX WITH HYPOECHOIC DEPOSITS WITH HYPERECHOIC AREAS

POSTERIOR ACOUSTIC SHADOW

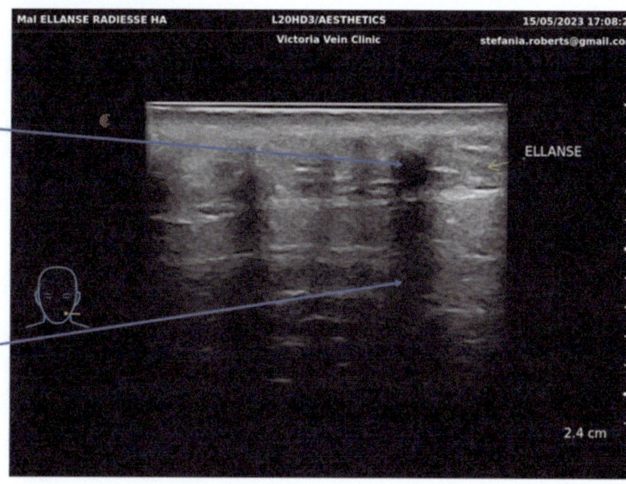

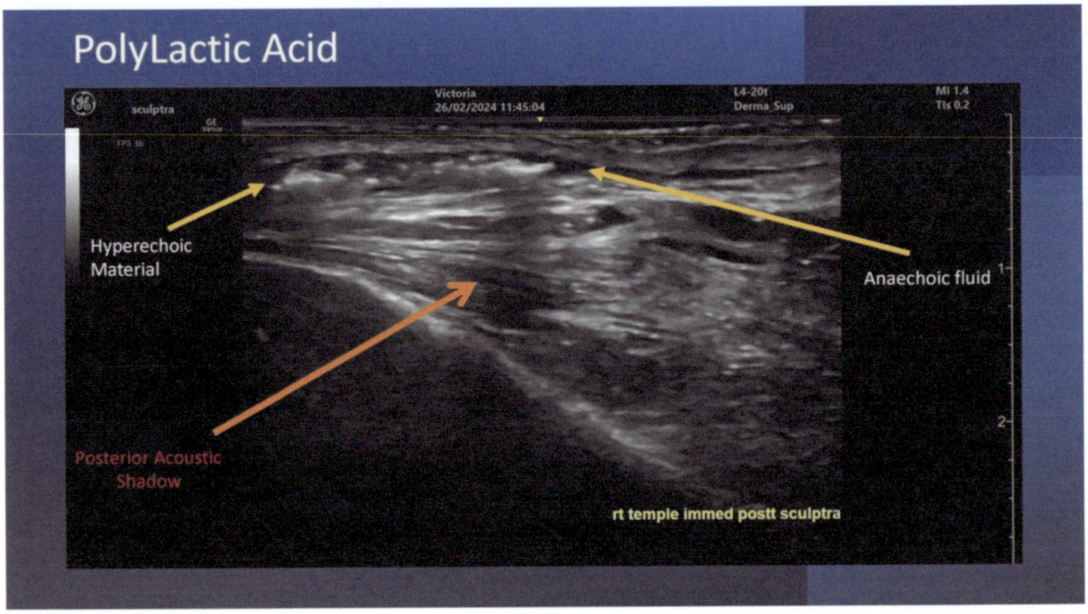

ULTRASOUND MORPHOLOGY OF CALCIUM HYDROXYAPETITE

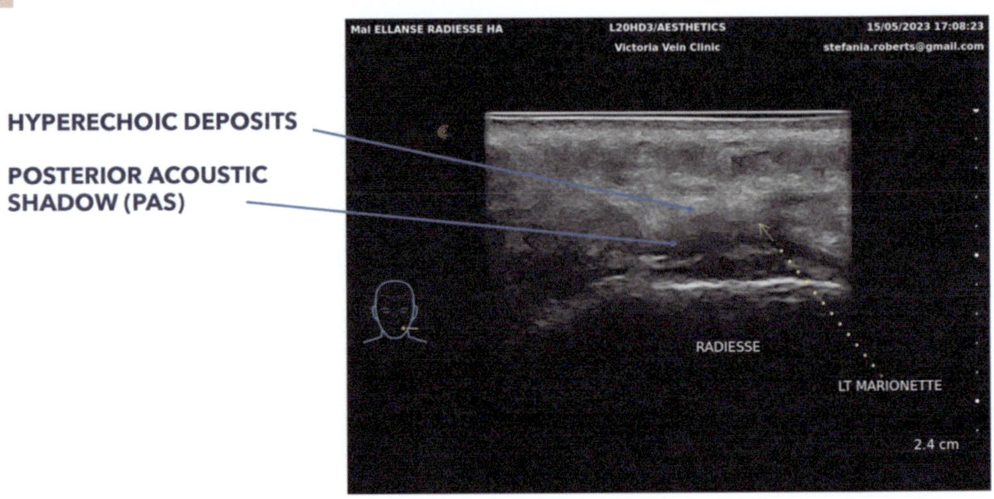

ULTRASOUND MORPHOLOGY OF PROFHILO – FACE IMMEDIATELY AND 14.5 HRS POST

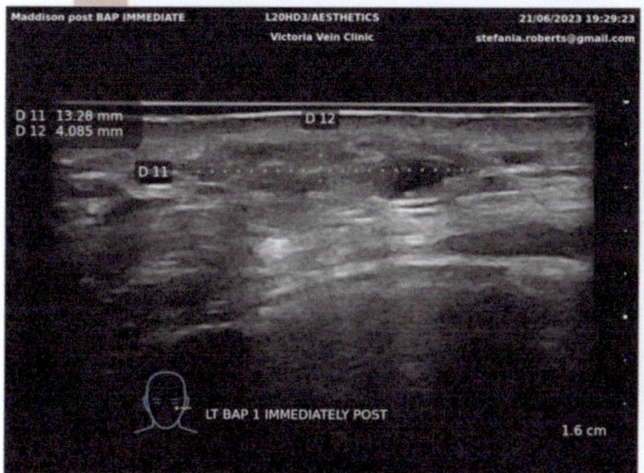

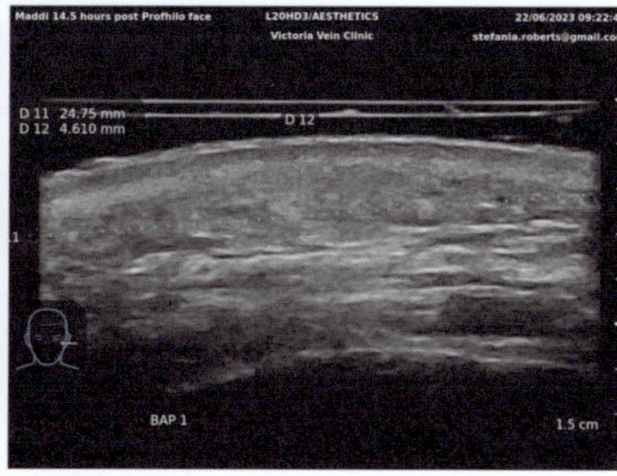

Diffuse
alternating hyperechoic and anechoic areas

heterogenous
ill-defined margins

ULTRASOUND MORPHOLOGY OF HYALURONIC ACID

ANECHOIC
HYPOECHOIC
NO HYPERECHOIC AREAS

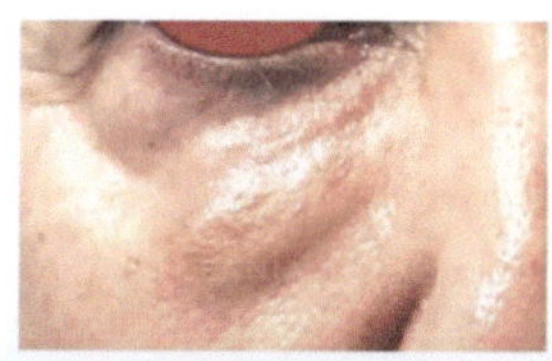

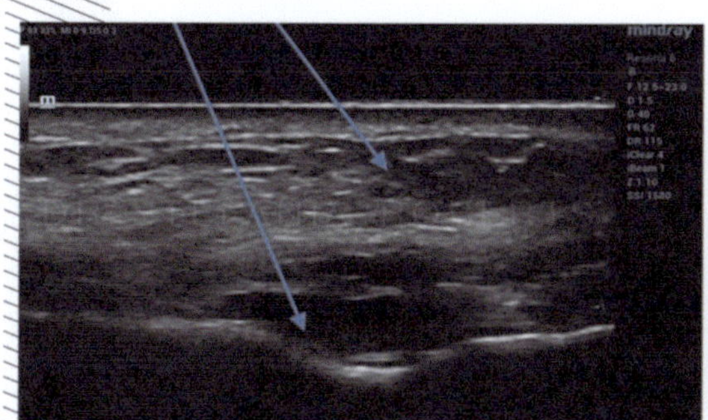

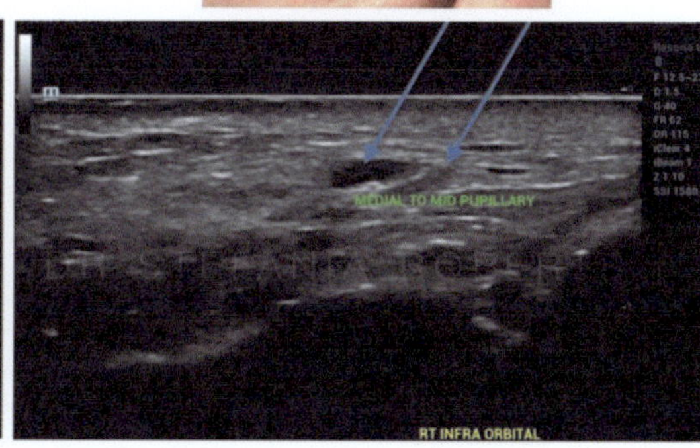

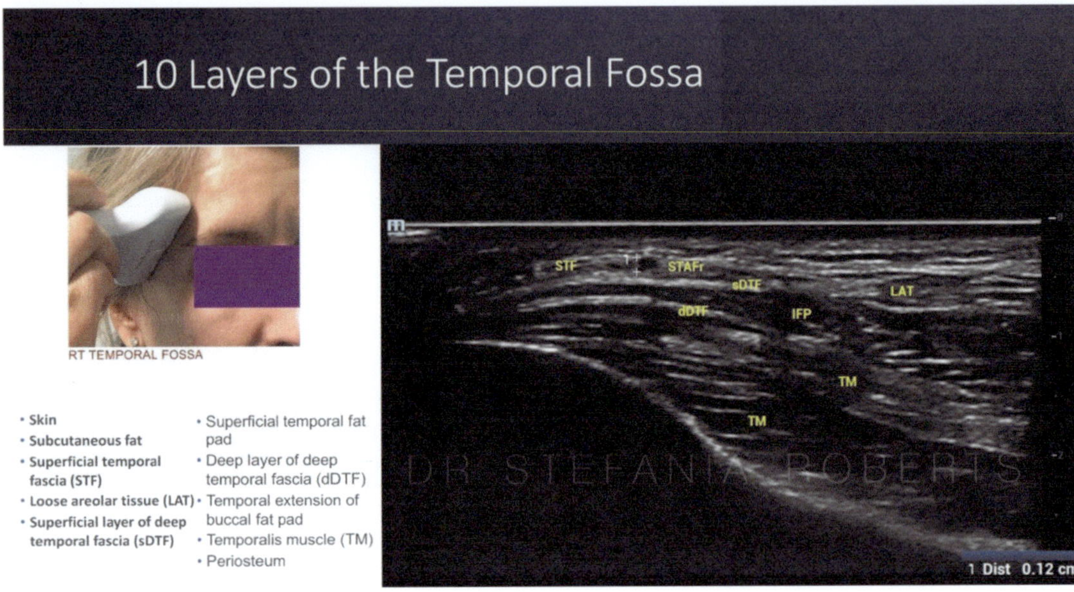
10 Layers of the Temporal Fossa
RT TEMPORAL FOSSA
• Skin
• Subcutaneous fat
• Superficial temporal fascia (STF)
• Loose areolar tissue (LAT)
• Superficial layer of deep temporal fascia (sDTF)
• Superficial temporal fat pad
• Deep layer of deep temporal fascia (dDTF)
• Temporal extension of buccal fat pad
• Temporalis muscle (TM)
• Periosteum
STF
STAFr
sDTF
dDTF
IFP
LAT
TM
TM
DR STEFANIA ROBERTS
1 Dist 0.12 cm

MIX
Papier aus verantwortungsvollen Quellen
Paper from responsible sources
FSC® C105338

If you have any concerns about our products, you can contact us on
ProductSafety@springernature.com

In case Publisher is established outside the EU, the EU authorized representative is:
Springer Nature Customer Service Center GmbH
Europaplatz 3, 69115 Heidelberg, Germany

Printed by Libri Plureos GmbH
in Hamburg, Germany